About the Author

Dr Marilyn Glenville PhD is the UK's leading nutritionist specialising in women's health. She obtained her doctorate from Cambridge University and is a fellow of the Royal Society of Medicine and a member of the Nutrition Society.

Dr Glenville is the former president of the Food and Health Forum at the Royal Society of Medicine and is patron of the Daisy Network, a premature menopause charity.

For more than 35 years, Dr Glenville has studied and practised nutrition, both in the UK and in the USA. She gives lectures and seminars throughout the world and appears regularly on radio and TV.

Dr Glenville has written 12 internationally best-selling books on women's healthcare which have sold over one million copies worldwide and have been translated into over 20 languages.

The books include;

Natural Solutions to the Menopause, Fat Around the Middle – and How to Lose it, Osteoporosis – How to Treat, Prevent and Reverse it, The Natural Health Bible for Women, Getting Pregnant Faster, Natural Solutions to PCOS, New Natural Alternatives to HRT, Healthy Eating for the Menopause, Natural Solutions to Infertility, The Nutritional Health Handbook for Women and *Overcoming PMS the Natural Way.*

Dr Glenville won the Best Nutrition Health Writer of the Year Award in 2009 and was awarded a place in the 2010 edition of *Who's Who* of famous people.

Dr Glenville runs clinics in Harley Street in London, Tunbridge Wells in Kent and Dublin, Galway and Cork in Ireland (see *Resources* page at back of book). Her website is www.marilynglenville.com.

Dedication

To all those men and women who are taking responsibility for their health.

Natural Alternatives
to Sugar

Dr Marilyn Glenville PhD

Natural Alternatives to Sugar

Dr Marilyn Glenville PhD

First published in the United Kingdom and Ireland in 2016 by Lifestyles Press

14 St John's Road, Tunbridge Wells, Kent TN4 9NP

Conceived, created and designed by Lifestyles Press 2016

Production Manager: Donna Gambazza, Lifestyles Press

Managing Designer: Sian Collins, www.siancollins-designer.com

British Library Cataloguing-in-Publication Data:

A CIP record for this book is available from the British Library

ISBN: 978-0-9935431-0-4

Typeset in Helvetica and ITC Garamond BT

Printed in UK

Notes: 1 tsp = 5ml

Disclaimer: The contents of this book are for information only and are intended to assist readers in identifying symptoms and conditions they may be experiencing. This book is not intended to be a substitute for taking proper medical advice and should not be relied upon in this way. Always consult a qualified doctor or health practitioner. The author and publisher cannot accept responsibility for illness arising out of the failure to seek medical advice from a doctor.

Contents

Introduction   9

Chapter 1:   The History of Sugar   11

Chapter 2:   What is Sugar?   15

Chapter 3:   What is the Problem with Sugar?   18

Chapter 4:   Sugar and Weight Gain   24

Chapter 5:   Sugar and Heart Disease   29

Chapter 6:   Sugar and Type 2 Diabetes   34

Chapter 7:   Sugar and Alzheimer's/Dementia   41

Chapter 8:   Sugar and Cancer   45

Chapter 9:   Sugar and Stress   48

Chapter 10:   Sugar and Ageing   53

Chapter 11:   What are the Alternatives?   55

Chapter 12:   Reading Food Labels   71

Chapter 13:   What to Eat to Control Sugar Cravings   74

Chapter 14:   The Five Day Sugar Detox   81

Chapter 15:   Should You Take Supplements?   91

Chapter 16:   Sugar-Free Recipes   101

Conclusion   140

Resources   143

References   145

Index   153

Acknowledgements

This has been an interesting book to write, as there is so much confusion on different websites about natural sweeteners. As well as looking at the information, it is important to know the source and then to weigh up and evaluate that information from different sources.

I have known about, and written about, the health risks of sugar since I wrote my first book in 1997 but it is only recently that it has really hit the media's attention and it is a subject I am very passionate about.

I would like to thank Jane Alexander for helping to make sure that this book is easy to read and to pick me up on parts where it got too technical, and not so practical, for the reader.

I would especially like to thank Helen Ford and Heather Leeson, two of my brilliant nutritionists who have supplied many of the recipes and I do hope you enjoy making and eating them.

I would also like to thank all the nutritionists who work with me in the UK (Anna Firth, Helen Ford, Sally Milne, Sharon Pitt and Lisa Smith) and those in Ireland headed by Heather Leeson (Ciara Wright, Sorcha Molloy, Helen Cassidy and Sarah Phillips).

Last but not least, my love goes to my family: Kriss, my husband, and my three children Matt (and his wife Hannah and their children Katie and Jack), Len and Chantell.

Introduction

Who doesn't love a sugary treat? From cupcakes to chocolate bars, from *The Great British Bake-Off* to Sunday afternoon crumpets and cake, we've been raised on the sweet stuff – sugar has been a lifelong treat for most of us. But now the tide is turning. Over the last few years, the media has been full of stories about the problems with sugar in our diet. Not to put too fine a point on it – we are putting our health, and even our lives, at risk with the overload of sugar in our diet.

However it seems there is still a great deal of confusion out there surrounding sugar:

- What do we mean by 'sugar'?
- What effects does sugar have on your health?
- If you do cut out or reduce sugar, what do you replace it with?

Again and again I am asked questions about sugar, both during consultations and in my talks. It is clear that people are still confused about the whole sugar issue: They want clear explanations of exactly why it is not good for their heath and what they can do about it. Hence this book.

I have been writing about the negative effects of sugar since my first book, *Natural Alternatives to HRT,* was published way back in 1997. But I always felt I was swimming against the tide. Back then, fat was seen as the bad guy and the emphasis was all on buying low fat and no fat foods. Fat was deemed to be fattening and the cause of heart disease and obesity.

This has always infuriated me.

Looking at the science and the research, this is a big fat lie that has been fed to us since the 1970s. In my opinion, it has contributed to our obesity and to the type 2 diabetes crisis we have, both in the UK and around most parts of the world. I will discuss how this lie began in the chapter on heart disease.

For now, let's be very clear. Sugar really is the enemy, not fat. If you want to live a healthy, happy, long life, it is absolutely essential that you get to grips with your sugar habit. The vast majority of people are addicted to sugar – there is evidence to show that your body reacts to it pretty much as it would to crack cocaine. The more sugar you have, the more your body craves, as it becomes de-sensitised. Sadly, food manufacturers, the media and even the health service have helped to ladle more and more sugar into your diet.

It's time to ditch the sugar and save your body, time to beat sugar cravings and learn how to eat real food, rather than empty, harmful calories. It is totally possible to reset your taste buds and recalibrate your body. The results are, quite frankly, extraordinary. Without sugar in your diet, you will feel better, brighter and clearer in mind and body. You will protect yourself from a large number of serious health conditions and many old aches, pains and niggling health concerns may disappear as if by magic.

Even moderate sugar intake on a regular basis can create or exacerbate a huge number of conditions; from fungal infections, mood swings, mucous production, low energy and libido, to brain fog and memory problems, inflammation and general lowered immunity.

Once your blood sugar levels stabilise, you will have more energy and you will undoubtedly sleep better. You will also notice a huge array of cosmetic effects – losing sugar will gain you a slimmer body and a clearer, brighter complexion.

What are you waiting for?

This book is your guide to living sugar-free or sugar-less. It will cover all the questions you have around sugar: its different forms, how it affects your health; the pros and cons of the various sugar substitutes. For those who are worrying about life without any sweetness, rest assured – I will also show you how you can still enjoy a touch of sweet – just without the health risks.

Let's get started...

CHAPTER 1

The History of Sugar

Know your enemy. In order to understand the role sugar plays in our lives, and how it has come to gain such prominence, we need a short history lesson. Knowledge is power. In this chapter, we will look at the grim history of sugar manufacture, which was based on that most iniquitous of practices – slavery.

Many years ago, sugar was a rare commodity. Our ancestors would have had no concept of refined sugar. In fact, refined sugars would have been completely absent in the diet of most people until very recently in our history.

Before the 20th century, it's highly unlikely that we would have eaten any more than a teaspoon of sugar per head, per year. Yes, just one teaspoon. Compare that with figures that estimate that in the US people can be consuming up to 46 teaspoons of sugar every day (and that's people who don't add sugar to their tea or coffee)[1].

Sugar was rationed in the UK in both world wars and in World War II it was restricted to 8oz (227g) per week. Let's put that into teaspoons - about 57 teaspoons per week! The National Diet and Nutrition Survey estimates that, here in the UK, we are consuming about 60g (15 teaspoons) of added sugar per day from all sources, but this is from people reporting, themselves, what they have eaten or drunk. It's not as extreme as the figures from the US but, even so, that's a lot of sugar.

Let's look at how much sugar we consume depending on our age.

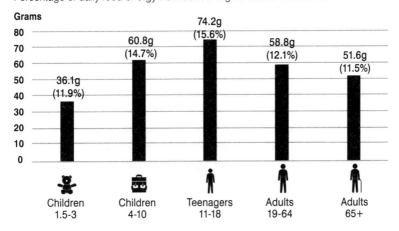

Daily added sugar intake, by age groups
Percentage of daily food energy from added sugars shown in brackets

Source: National Diet & Nutrition Survey, rolling programme 2008-12

So what are the origins of our sugar fix? Historians can't pin down the exact date of the first extraction of sugar from sugar cane but it was likely to have been around 10,000 years ago on the Polynesian islands in the Pacific Ocean. Before they started extracting sugar, people would just pick the cane and eat it raw to get the sweet taste (now that really was eating sugar as a wholefood in its natural state).

Sugar cane was taken to India and processed into a powder that was used to sweeten food. However, it was also considered a medicine. By 600 BC, sugar refining had reached Persia and by 400 BC, Alexander the Great transplanted the sugar cane to Greece.

Sugar cane was then cultivated in Mediterranean regions including Spain and Portugal. It was a highly profitable crop, as its novelty gave it great value. Sugar was expensive, very expensive, a luxury food that only the rich could afford.

It was Columbus who realised that the West Indies had the ideal climate for growing sugar cane and so production in the Mediterranean waned.

At first, the sugar canes were farmed by local people in the West Indies but, as demand increased and production grew rapidly, sugar became big business. More workers were needed. This was when slaves were brought over from Africa to work on the sugar plantations.

In 1627, 50 British settlers landed in Barbados, aiming to transform the land for farming. They brought their own workers with them, who were classed as indentured labourers. This meant that they agreed to work for their employer for a set number of years (usually five), during which they would learn a skill and after which they would be freed.

The farming initially included cotton, tobacco and indigo. Indigo was a plant which produced dyes ranging from deep red to deep blue - the dyes were very expensive.

The settlers then decided to experiment and grow a new crop - sugar. This had been brought over from New Guinea by the Portuguese. However, instead of using indentured labourers, they started using African slaves. The work needed to produce sugar from sugar cane was back-breaking, labour-intensive work. The moment sugar cane is harvested it starts to spoil, so it had to be moved quickly to the next part of the process, which meant the African slaves had to labour throughout the night.

They used windmills to process the sugar cane. Once again, if the juice was not processed into granules quickly enough it would ferment and spoil.

Once processed, the sugar was then shipped to Europe.

African slaves arriving in Barbados had a life expectancy of seven years, thanks to the brutal system of working.

Because sugar was such a lucrative commodity, this model of working was transplanted to other Caribbean islands. Sugar was so profitable that it was often referred to as 'white gold' - having a sugar plantation was the equivalent of owning a gold mine.

In contrast to indentured labourers, slaves were deemed to be 'property' and, therefore, were 'owned' by the masters. Researchers have found 'slave codes' in British colonies - sets of laws which defined the statuses of slaves and the rights and responsibilities of slave owners.

The whole system was based on terror. Slaves were forbidden from leaving the owner's property and, if they ran away, they were likely to receive a death penalty. They were forbidden from learning to read and write, whipping and punishment were commonplace and no slave was allowed to work for pay or to keep their own livestock or crops. If a slave were killed by an 'owner', no punishment would occur.

This system continued for 200 years because it generated so much wealth. It also had a huge and positive impact on the British economy as large docks, such as the West India Dock in London, were built to bring the sugar in quickly.

In 1807, the transatlantic slave trade was outlawed, meaning that slaves could not be transported, but this did not abolish slavery.

British slave owners then looked elsewhere and started to buy up Dutch plantations in Guyana. These plantations grew cotton and coffee and were already worked by slaves, so none needed to be transported. But the British saw bigger profits in sugar and they realised that one particular island, called Demerara, had good, fertile soil. They saw that they could make even bigger profits here than anywhere else in the Caribbean. By 1820, British sugar plantations in Guyana were worked by about 100,000 slaves.

1833 marked the abolition of slavery. However, the British Government had to compensate the slave owners £20 million (equivalent to £17 billion in today's money). A national commission, called the Slave Compensation Commission, was established to settle the compensation. In Britain 3,000 slave owners owned 50 per cent of the slaves and, come abolition, there were 800,000 slaves. However, even after abolition was declared, the slaves still had to work unpaid for another six years.

The compensation that was paid made many former slave owners in Britain very wealthy and that money was invested in industry, finance and the railways. We should never forget that sugar and slavery made Britain prosperous.

When sugar was initially imported into the UK it was expensive, heavily taxed and well out of the reach of most people. Those people who could afford it often bought it as a cone from which they chipped off pieces using 'nippers', which looked like a pair of pincers. Alternatively, they bought it in lump form.

In the 19th century, Napoleon blocked the trade routes and stopped sugar being imported by sea. In the UK it was found that sugar could be extracted not just from sugar cane but also from sugar beets. However, at that time, it was not possible to extract as much sugar from the beet as could be obtained from the cane. Even today, with modern extraction processes, the amount of sugar obtained from cane is six times higher than from beets.

After the Napoleonic Wars ended, the trade routes opened again. In 1874, William Gladstone, the UK Prime Minister, removed the tax from sugar, putting it within the reach of more people. But the more easily available sugar became, the more people wanted it and demand kept increasing. Why? Because sugar is highly addictive.

Nowadays, Brazil, India and the European Union are the top three producers of sugar. In the UK, sugar makes up a colossal 12 per cent (or more) of the average daily diet, while children and teenagers are eating over 15 per cent.

In the next chapter, we'll take a closer look at what we actually mean by 'sugar'.

CHAPTER 2

What is Sugar?

When most of us think about sugar, we visualise the white crystals you find in the sugar bowl, either loose as granules or formed into sugar cubes. In fact, this is just one type of sugar, known as sucrose. 'Sugar' is a collective term for any soluble sweet-tasting carbohydrate. Generally, the different kinds of sugars end in -ose. So sucrose, lactose, fructose, glucose, maltose and dextrose would all be classed as sugar.

Sucrose is usually made from either sugar cane or sugar beet and arrives in our homes in various different forms; for example, granulated sugar, table sugar, caster sugar, icing sugar or sugar cubes (in which the crystals are held together with sugar syrup). Sugar can also be brown in colour, as in turbinado, muscovado and demerara sugars, in which some of the molasses have been retained, giving the sugar a brown colour. Molasses are the by-product of the process used to extract the sugar from the cane or beet.

There are also liquid sugars, which are just sugar granules dissolved in water, plus syrups and treacles, which can be used to make sweets and as ingredients in baked foods.

Sugar alcohols (polyols) like xylitol, sorbitol and erythritol are also available.

In addition, there are a host of artificial sweeteners which are used as alternatives to sugar. I will discuss all of these later in the book.

We will also look at whether the more 'natural' choices of sweeteners are actually healthful - or just as bad as 'normal' sugar.

As I've already said, sugar is a carbohydrate. Carbohydrates provide energy for your body, including your brain and nervous system. An enzyme called amylase breaks down carbohydrates, which are then utilised by your body. Carbohydrates are classified as either simple or complex, depending on their chemical structure. Complex carbohydrates are made up of three or more simple sugars - for example, starchy vegetables such as potatoes; beans, lentil and pulses; and wholegrain foods such as oatmeal, wholewheat pasta and wholegrain bread. It takes your body longer to break down the sugars in these, so they give you longer-lasting energy.

Simple carbohydrates fall into two categories: Monosaccharides (one sugar molecule) and disaccharides (two sugar molecules).

Where the different sugars are found

Glucose: Found in all carbohydrates. This is the form that your body uses for energy (also called dextrose). Your blood sugar level is the amount of glucose in your blood.

Fructose: Fruit sugar found in fruits and vegetables.

Galactose: Found in milk, fruits and vegetables.

Sucrose: Made from sugar cane or beet.

Lactose: Milk sugar found in milk products.

Maltose: Made from grains such as barley.

The disaccharides are made up of two sugar molecules, so sucrose is made up of glucose (50 per cent) and fructose (50 per cent) which are bound together and then split again as you digest the sucrose. Lactose is broken down into glucose (50 per cent) and galactose (50 per cent) and maltose into two glucose molecules (50 per cent each).

Why am I giving so much information on the chemical components of sugar? You might think the actual form sugar comes in doesn't really matter, but it does. The effect various forms of sugar have on your body when you digest them is what is causing so much upset in the media and so much disagreement among experts. Some critics claim that all sugar is the same - these are probably the people who think that all calories are equal or that fat makes us fat. It's simply not true. The chemical composition of the various sugars affects how you absorb them, what they do to your appetite and also what they do to your metabolism. Not all sugars are created equal - different sugars will affect your weight, your waistline and, ultimately, your health in different ways.

I will discuss other forms of sweeteners later in the book but, for now, I would just like to draw your attention to two in particular.

Maltodextrin

You will often see this ingredient listed on food products and in supplements like probiotics. It is a synthetic polysaccharide, made up of glucose molecules, and is produced by the partial hydrolysis of starch (such as rice, corn or potato starch).

Maltodextrin is quickly digested: Because it is made up of glucose molecules, it is absorbed as rapidly as glucose and has a high glycaemic index.

As you'll know if you've read my previous books, the Glycaemic Index (GI) is a ranking of carbohydrate-containing foods based on the overall effect they have on your blood glucose levels. Slowly absorbed foods have a low GI rating, while foods that are more quickly absorbed have a higher rating. Foods are given a GI number according to their effect on blood glucose levels. Glucose is used as a standard reference (GI 100) and other foods are measured against this.

So it is not good that it has a high GI but recent research suggests that maltodextrin may suppress the anti-microbial defense mechanisms in your digestive system, as it promoted Salmonella survival in a mice study and could also make you more prone to inflammation[2].

High fructose corn syrup (HFCS)

High fructose corn syrup deserves a special mention as you will no doubt have seen the media give a lot of attention to this type of sugar. HFCS is a mixture of glucose and fructose but is about 30 per cent cheaper than regular table sugar (sucrose). It is converted from corn and can contain up to 90 per cent fructose. It is most widely used in America, where regular sugar costs more than in other parts of the world. There are also subsidies on corn, so HFCS is a much cheaper alternative and, hence, used much more widely. HFCS is produced by first making corn starch from corn and then refining the starch into corn syrup. Enzymes are then added to the syrup to change a percentage of the glucose into fructose. In the UK, you may find it labelled as glucose-fructose or fructose-glucose syrup on ingredient lists. There are serious health concerns about HFCS, which I will cover in the next chapter.

So now you know what sugar actually is. Let's look next at why it is so bad for us. What is the problem with sugar?

CHAPTER 3

What is the Problem with Sugar?

In a nutshell, sugar in any form (sucrose, fructose and so on) provides empty calories. In other words, it has no nutritional value whatsoever. It is important to clarify that this refers to the refined sugar added to your food and drink and not to the naturally-occurring sugar in certain foods such as fruit, vegetables and grains.

The NHS says that added sugar can make up to ten per cent of your daily calorie intake. That means 50g (12.5 teaspoons) a day for women and 70g (17.5 teaspoons a day for men). That is a *lot* of sugar. I have to say I totally disagree with this advice. It's like saying that if you didn't eat any foods containing added sugar you could safely add 12.5 teaspoons of sugar to your tea or coffee in a day. The World Health Organisation (WHO) wants to limit added sugar (including honey) to just six teaspoons a day for both men and women.

It's a step in the right direction but, in my opinion (and that of a huge number of nutritional experts and medical doctors), you don't need *any* added sugar at all. Sugar is a carbohydrate and we get quite enough carbohydrates from all the other foods that we eat. However, the food industry doesn't want us to know that. They seek to keep profits at the maximum and so sugar levels are kept high.

Controversy reared up in 2014 when it was shown that five out of the eight members on the Scientific Advisory Committee on Nutrition (SACN) were being funded by sugar or food companies. SACN is the committee that has written a report on sugar and health. How can its members possibly be impartial when they have such very close relationships with the food industries that want to keep sugar consumption high?

Let me reiterate so it's totally clear: The food industry does not want us to lower our intake of sugar. The more sugar we eat, the more sugar we want and, hence, the more sugar-laden food products we will buy. The seemingly independent sounding British Nutrition Foundation has an interesting list of Member Companies in their Annual Report and Accounts. These Member Companies include Coca Cola, British Sugar, Heinz, Kellogg's, McDonald's, Pepsi, United Biscuits and Weetabix - all of which use a high proportion of sugars and sweeteners in their products[3].

Also, the UK's Change4Life 'Sugar Swaps' campaign involves Coca-Cola offering artificially sweetened drinks in place of their sugared soft drinks. Is this a healthy swap? Not in my opinion. You will find out why in the alternative sweeteners section of this book.

On the other side of the coin, as well as the WHO wanting to limit sugar, the UK Government's Chief Medical Officer has suggested that a sugar tax needs to be added to certain foods.

It is estimated that adding seven pence to the price of a can of soft drink would generate £1 billion a year and that it might reduce obesity by 200,000 people, saving the NHS £15 million a year.

The SACN report on carbohydrates, published in July 2015, suggests that no more than five per cent of our daily food should be taken as sugar; that equates to 25g (five teaspoons) for women and 35g (eight teaspoons) for men. So just one fizzy soft drink would put you over their limit.

A report released in October 2015 by Public Health England, entitled *Sugar Reduction: The Evidence for Action* says that we should get no more than five per cent of our energy intake from sugar. They are suggesting that if people reduced their sugar intake, it would save 77,000 lives. The report has called for a tax of 20 per cent on sugary foods and drinks (not just drinks). This report said that adults are consuming more than twice the recommended limit and teenagers three times more.

This report also recommends that there should be a clamp down on discount offers on sugary foods and drinks, such as buy one get one free, and also a significant reduction in the advertising of high sugar food and drink to children. There is a marketing spend of £256 million in the UK each year to advertise these foods and drinks to us and parents do find it hard to say no to their children when a cereal, for instance, is endorsed by a popular cartoon character.

We have already seen in Chapter 1 how our consumption of sugar has changed and increased over the centuries. The problem is that sugar is not just found in the obvious sweet foods that you eat (for example, cakes, sweets, chocolate) but it is also 'hidden' in unlikely places, including savoury foods such as tomato ketchup, mayonnaise and salad dressing.

Our sugar consumption has increased because sugar is now cheap and can be added to many different foods, sweet and savoury. Plus it tastes good. We are born with a sweet tooth so we are naturally drawn to sweet food. Breast milk is very sweet and it is thought that this natural attraction to sweetness has evolutionary advantages. Sweetness indicates that a food has more calories and, hence, is energy dense. Energy-rich foods would have been vital for our survival in the past. Also sweet tastes tend to be a good indicator that a food is safe to eat - bitter tasting foods are more likely to be toxic and would be avoided.

However, this natural tendency toward sweeter foods means that sugar is often added to a huge variety of different foods, in order to make them taste more appealing, so we eat more of them.

The health consequences of this are enormous, as you will see in the following chapters, but everyone already connects eating too much sugar with dental decay. And the problem with sugar rotting teeth is that it is now the number one reason that children are admitted to hospital to have their teeth removed. Twenty six thousand primary school age children are now admitted to hospital each year to have teeth extracted and it is costing the NHS £30 million a year.

Quite apart from our inborn preference for sweet foods, there is another problem around sugar. Research indicates quite clearly that it has an addictive quality.

Research on rats who were induced to become sugar-bingers showed signs of opiate-like withdrawal when their sugar was removed. Bear in mind that both heroin and cocaine are opiates. The rats got the shakes and tremors when the sugar was withdrawn. When sugar was introduced again two weeks later, the rats consumed 23 per cent more than they had before[4].

Other research on rats has shown that, when the animals were allowed to choose freely between highly sweetened water and intravenous cocaine, 94 per cent preferred the sweet drink. The researchers concluded that 'intense sweetness can surpass cocaine reward… The supranormal stimulation of these receptors by sugar-rich diets, such as those now widely available in modern societies, would generate a supranormal reward signal in the brain, with the potential to override self-control mechanisms and thus to lead to addiction'[5]. So sugar is actually more addictive than cocaine!

Further research, this time on humans at the Harvard Medical School, found similar results. The researchers gave 12 overweight men one of two milkshakes. One milkshake had a high glycaemic index (GI) and the other low, but both tasted the same and contained the same amount of calories. High glycaemic index foods cause a rapid rise and then a slump in blood sugar.

The milkshakes were given on different days and four hours after the men had the high GI milkshake they were hungrier than those who had the low GI drink. The researchers also watched what happened in the brain in response to the high GI and low GI milkshakes on an MRI scan.

The results were very interesting because the images after the high GI milkshake showed intense activity of a structure in the brain called the nucleus accumbens, which is associated with pleasure eating, reward and craving. The same 'lighting up' of this area of the brain can be seen after people use cocaine and heroin.

The researchers suggest that this supports the argument that food can be addictive and that we eat not just for our survival and daily energy needs[6].

The more you eat, the more you want. Some patients of mine have called themselves 'carboholics' because they feel they are addicted to carbohydrates like white flour and sugar, just as if they were an alcoholic. They have a fair point.

Are you addicted to sugar?

The American Psychiatric Association has a manual entitled the *Diagnostic and Statistical Manual of Mental Disorders* and it suggests that the following list indicates the type of behaviours that could indicate an addiction. Run through this list and look at your behaviour over the last year, when it comes to eating sugar and sugary foods.

- Tolerance.
- Withdrawal.
- The substance is often taken in larger amounts than intended.
- A persistent desire or unsuccessful efforts to cut down substance use.
- A great deal of time is spent in activities necessary to obtain the substance.
- Important activities are given up or reduced because of substance use.
- Substance use is continued despite knowledge of having a persistent or recurrent physical or psychological problem that is likely to have been caused or exacerbated by the substance.

There is another version called *The Yale Food Addiction Scale* which asks the questions in a slightly different way. Again, think of the questions in the context of eating sugar and sugary foods.

Answer yes or no to the following seven statements:

1. I eat certain foods even if I am no longer hungry.
2. I feel sluggish or fatigued from overeating.
3. My behaviour with respect to food causes me distress.
4. I have had physical withdrawal symptoms, such as agitation and anxiety, when I cut down on certain foods (not including coffee and tea).
5. I have spent time dealing with negative feelings from overeating, instead of spending time on family, friends, work or recreation.
6. I am consuming the same types or amounts of food, despite significant emotional or physical problems related to my eating.
7. Over time, I have found that I need to eat more and more to get the feeling I want, such as reduced negative emotions or increased pleasure.

If you answered 'yes' (and this happens more than three times a week) to the first five, and simply 'yes' to the other two, you need to take a long look at your eating habits, as it is very likely you do have a problem with sugar.

High Fructose Corn Syrup (HFCS)/Fructose

I mentioned this type of sweetener in the last chapter. It is very popular in America because it is cheaper to use than sugar and the USA has an abundance of corn with which to make HFCS. It is not used as much in the UK but, as I've previously mentioned, it does sometimes crop up - it will appear on labels as 'glucose-fructose syrup' or 'fructose-glucose syrup'.

However, I will now look more closely at the health issues linked to HFCS. I will also talk about fructose, which is widely used in the UK, because the effects on our bodies are very similar.

The fructose we are discussing here is the white, refined powdered fructose that can be bought as a sweetener and which can be added as an ingredient in foods, drinks and even food supplements.

It was first thought that fructose could be a useful substitute for sucrose (table sugar) and might be helpful for diabetes because it does not cause the release of insulin.

However, because fructose does not use insulin to remove it from your bloodstream, your liver has to metabolise it on its own. Fructose triggers lipogenesis (the production of fats, e.g. cholesterol and triglycerides) in your liver which can, in turn, lead to 'fatty liver' and liver damage but also to an increased risk of heart disease. High levels of triglycerides are also associated with type 2 diabetes so it's ironic that many people switch to fructose instead of sucrose in an attempt to stop insulin spikes.

The metabolism of fructose is twice as fast as glucose metabolism, so the toll on your body is harder.

In addition, fructose suppresses the hormone leptin, which is the hormone that lets you know when you are full. When leptin is suppressed it means you have far less control over your appetite because you will still feel hungry.

So what about fructose in fruit? Does this mean we should be avoiding fruit? Not at all. HFCS and refined fructose are known as 'unbound' or 'free' but when the fructose is contained within fruit it is bound up with the vitamins and minerals, fibre, fatty acids and other sugars within that food so it does not affect your liver in the same way.

Research comparing the effect of fructose-sweetened drinks with glucose-sweetened drinks on obese people, found that those who had the fructose-sweetened drinks with their meals had triglyceride levels 200 per cent higher than those who drank the glucose-sweetened drinks with their food[7].

So, sugar is highly addictive and can have a detrimental effect on your health. Over the next few chapters, we will look in more detail at exactly how far it can impact your health and wellbeing. We'll start with how sugar can contribute to weight gain.

CHAPTER 4

Sugar and Weight Gain

Fat is fattening? No. It's nonsense; a big fat diet lie. Please forget the myth that fat is fattening; it is sugar and refined carbohydrates that make you fat. Sugar, as I've already said, is nothing more than empty calories - it gives you no nutritional value at all. Worse than that, because sugar is devoid of nutrients, your body has to use other nutrients stored in your system in order to digest the sugar. So, not only are you getting absolutely no vital vitamins and minerals from the sugar, but your body is also losing valuable nutrients just by eating it. Hence, sugar causes a double whammy on the nutritional front and can actually create nutritional deficiencies.

For many decades, gaining and losing weight had always been considered to be about calories. However, not all calories are equal. It all depends on the form that the calories take, which determines whether they are going to cause a problem with weight gain or not.

To explain how sugar makes you gain weight, it is useful to know what happens in your body as you eat and, in particular, what happens when you consume sugary foods or drinks.

When you eat, your food is broken down by digestion into glucose (sugar) and absorbed through the walls of your small intestines. It's perfectly natural to have a high level of glucose in your blood after eating. Your pancreas then releases the hormone insulin to move the glucose (sugar) from your blood, into your cells, to be used for energy. If you have taken in more sugar than your body needs for energy, your body will store it. The glucose is changed into glycogen and stored in your liver and muscles to be used later. The glucose level in your blood should then return to a normal level.

The role of insulin

When you eat sugar or sugary foods, the food is digested very quickly and you will have much higher levels of glucose in your blood which, in turn, will require more insulin to be released by your pancreas. Think of insulin as the 'fat storing hormone' of your body. When it is released, it directs the energy from your food into storage. So the more insulin you produce the more your food is likely to be stored as fat. A small amount is stored as glycogen but the majority is stored as fat.

Unfortunately, when your insulin levels are high, your body doesn't use fat for fuel; it uses the glucose in your blood instead. So when insulin is being produced, you won't lose weight; your body will cling onto your fat stores.

Your body has a brilliant mechanism for keeping your blood sugar in balance:

- When your blood sugar level rises too high, your body produces more insulin to balance it.

- When your blood sugar level is too low, the hormones adrenaline and cortisol are released from the adrenal glands and glucagon is produced from the pancreas. Glucagon works in the opposite way to insulin and increases blood glucose, by encouraging the liver to turn some of its glycogen stores into glucose.

As we saw in the last chapter, insulin also blocks the production of a hormone called leptin. This hormone is often called the 'hunger hormone' because it lets your brain know that you are full.

Leptin is produced by your fat cells and its job is to warn you that you have had enough to eat - it's responsible for that satisfied feeling. So, you might think that, the more fat you have, the better the effect would be, as you would be producing even more leptin. Unfortunately, if your body fat percentage is raised too high, you can become leptin resistant. This means that your body will not register the effects of this hormone and consequently you will end up feeling less satisfied with the amount of food you are eating.

It is thought that fructose worsens this effect. We will discuss this later in the book.

In addition, cortisol (the hormone that is released along with adrenaline when your blood sugar drops) prevents leptin from decreasing your appetite and keeping your weight under control.

Not getting enough sleep also makes you produce less leptin. In addition, lack of sleep can cause you to produce more of the 'hunger hormone' ghrelin (which is released by your stomach). Lack of sleep also makes you become insulin resistant and that can start after only one night of sleeping for four hours[8]. If that lack of sleep carries on over six nights, it will reduce your body's ability to respond to insulin by 30 per cent[9].

Fat around the middle

Too much sugar and sugary foods make you gain weight but they also can make you gain weight in a certain part of your body. I have written a very popular book called *Fat around the Middle* on exactly this issue. The problem is that people, and in particular women, are changing shape.

The classic woman's figure was pear-shaped, the hourglass figure typified by Marilyn Monroe. However, over recent years, women have become more apple-shaped, which has traditionally been associated with male weight gain.

The chart below shows how much women's shapes have changed over the years.

Figures published in 2004 showed that between 1951 and 2004, women's waists increased by 6.5in (16.5cm).

However, compare the other changes in height, bust and hips.

	1951	2004	Difference
Height	5ft 3in	5ft 4.5in	1.5in
Bust	37in	38.5in	1.5in
Hips	39in	40.5in	1.5in
Waist	27.5in	34in	6.5in

Source: National Sizing Survey

Women have become taller and larger around the hips by 1.5 inches (3.8cms) but have become a massive 6.5 inches larger around the waist.

Men have also seen an increase in waist measurement but only by 1.5 inches (3.8cms).

What is causing this massive weight gain around the middle of the body? It's the effect of cortisol being released when your blood sugar drops. The message sent to your body from high insulin levels as your blood sugar rises is to store your food as fat. Then again, when your blood sugar drops, cortisol is released and the message this hormone sends out is more of the same: store that fat around your middle.

This is a protective mechanism and it's understandable why your body would do it but, sadly, it's not remotely healthy. Quite apart from the effect this fat has on your health, it's also a source of great misery to many people, particularly women. Clothes don't fit properly or look as good; nobody likes the look of a wodge of weight sitting around the middle. 'I look pregnant' is a common complaint from my patients who suffer from 'fat around the middle'.

Your body has been designed primarily to react quickly to danger. This was crucial years ago when you needed to be on constant alert so that you could run or fight for survival.

This fight or flight response is incredible - it provides instant energy for five to ten minutes, allowing you to react quickly in order to save your life.

When your brain thinks your life is in danger it stimulates the release of the stress hormones adrenaline and cortisol.

These hormones are still released nowadays from the stresses and strains of everyday life such as work and relationships. Your body often doesn't recognise the difference between a life-threatening situation and one of emotional stress. However, as we have seen above, stress hormones are also released according to your pattern of eating; for example, from eating too much sugar and sugary foods.

Normally, when faced with a life or death situation when adrenaline and cortisol are released, you would expend a large amount of energy to run away or to turn and fight. However, obviously, when stress hormones are released from the blood sugar roller coaster, there is no need to fight or run, so you are not using up that available energy. All the extra energy released (fat and glucose) when your blood sugar drops is then deposited as fat. Where is it stored? In the main, it sits around your middle.

Your body places fat here because it is close to your liver, where it can be converted back into energy as quickly as possible when needed. If it's stored down on your hips or thighs, it's simply too far away to be reached swiftly in an emergency. Think of it as having a protective cushion around your middle. It's your body's equivalent of keeping your foot hovering over the brake pedal - it's on high alert, thinking there could be a life or death situation at any minute and so it needs a handy energy store to call on should you need to run or fight for your life. But, of course, your life is not in danger. Your body only thinks it might be because of the message it is being given from the cortisol being released from your roller coaster of blood sugar swings.

Not only will you gain weight from this but you will also have cravings for more sugar and sweet foods and a general increase in appetite because your body wants to make sure it always has a good supply of energy in case it needs to call on it.

Cephalic phase insulin release

This sounds like a mouthful but it's a very interesting process that happens in your body: quite probably you have not heard much about it.

Even before you eat, just thinking about food - its taste, texture and smell - causes your brain to start to prepare your body for the idea of eating. If your brain thinks that the food is going to be very sugary it will stimulate your pancreas to release more insulin, even before you have put the food in your mouth.

It is basically the *anticipation* of food preparing your body for digestion that can cause the increased release of insulin. It can also make you overeat if you smell your favourite meal. Even the feel of food in your mouth or thoughts related to that food (such as memories/previous experiences of eating it) will send signals for your body to release stomach acid in preparation for the food to be swallowed.

Just putting food on your tongue can elicit this cephalic phase insulin release. In one study, researchers asked volunteers to swill different liquids around their mouths and then spit them out again, so they did not swallow them. Both water containing sugar and one containing artificial sweeteners caused a significant increase in blood levels of insulin[10].

The memories of how you have eaten in the past can trigger the release of too much insulin, especially if you had a sweet tooth.

It really does sound as if your body chemistry is against you, doesn't it? But the good news is that, once you have made the changes suggested in this book, your body can be retrained not to react in the old way, as it anticipates the intake of less sugary food, creating a better balance with your blood sugar.

In the next chapter, we'll look at how sugar can play a leading role in causing heart disease.

CHAPTER 5

Sugar and Heart Disease

The prevailing wisdom for many years has been that it is fat that causes heart disease; hence we have all been led into buying low-fat and no-fat foods. As I have said previously, this is a complete myth: It is sugar and foods that are broken down into sugar quickly (like refined carbohydrates, white bread, white rice and so forth) that are the culprits.

How did this lie start? Well, it all began with rabbits!

In 1913, a Russian researcher called Nikolaj Nikolajewitsch Anitschkow showed that when rabbits were fed a cholesterol-laden diet they developed plaque in the arteries (atherosclerosis). He also said that the amount of cholesterol given to the rabbits was directly proportional to the degree of atherosclerosis formation. The greater the amount of cholesterol the rabbits were given, the worse the plaque formation. But, and this is an enormous but, rabbits do not normally eat any foods containing cholesterol. Only animal foods contain cholesterol. Rabbits are vegetarians, so their bodies are not designed to deal with cholesterol[11].

So the myth started that excess cholesterol in the arteries causes plaque, which is due to excess cholesterol in the blood, which is due to fatty foods containing cholesterol in the diet.

Other studies that followed used carnivorous animals fed in the same cholesterol-laden way as the rabbits, but they failed to show that fatty deposits of plaque built up in the arteries.

However, the theory that fatty food causes heart disease was further perpetuated by an American physiologist called Ancel Keys who, in 1970, reported that there was a higher incidence of heart disease in countries with a higher intake of saturated fats[12].

Keys looked at data from seven countries to come to this conclusion. However, seven countries is not a large number and also, more crucially, he omitted a number of European countries, such as France. France is important for what is known as the 'French Paradox'. The French have a high intake of fatty foods but a low rate of heart disease.

In 1977, avoiding or reducing fat became government policy in the US, with the introduction of the McGovern dietary guidelines. In 1983, the UK followed suit.

I have been writing about our erroneous perceptions on the question of sugar and fat in our diets since 1997 and have included warnings in my previous books about sugar. However, it is not always easy to change something that has been churned out like a mantra for so many years, namely that fat causes heart disease. I remember a few years back giving a talk at the Royal Society of Medicine on this very subject and, during question time, a GP said that he had been trying to get the message across to his patients that, in fact, sugar and refined carbohydrates were the culprits. However, the other doctors in his practice told him that if he did not toe the party line with the 'fat is bad' concept, he would be asked to leave.

Changing people's long-held beliefs that fat is bad is not going to be easy, even in the light of new research. It is like trying to turn round a huge ocean liner; the process is going to be very slow and some experts will still not want to relinquish their old beliefs.

Recent research is showing why it's imperative that this belief changes and needs to change quickly. We already have an obesity and type 2 diabetes crisis in the UK, just as many other countries do. This will only get worse if the wrong advice continues to be given. Over the last 30 years in the UK, obesity rates have trebled, with 65 per cent of adults being overweight or obese. Meanwhile, the proportion of fats in our diet has decreased by six per cent. If you needed any more proof that fat is not the enemy, there it is.

Researchers have looked at whether increasing or decreasing dairy foods could have any effect on blood pressure, cholesterol, triglycerides, glucose, insulin and C-reactive protein, a marker of inflammation. The answer is no; there was no change in any of those readings in either those people who increased or those who decreased their dairy food consumption[13].

In 2015, a study in the *British Medical Journal, Open Heart*, showed evidence that dietary recommendations to reduce fat to less than a third of total energy intake had been introduced to 220 million people in the US in 1970 and to 56 million in the UK by 1983, without the supporting evidence from randomised controlled trials[14].

The connection between sugar and heart disease

We now know that fat does not cause heart disease. So where does the sugar connection come in?

Once again, it all comes down to insulin, the hormone released when your blood sugar rises. When you have a meal, insulin normally sends a signal to your liver not to release fats into your bloodstream because your body is dealing with fat from the meal.

However, if you are living on that roller coaster of blood sugar swings, as I've already explained, too much insulin is being released too often and your liver then ignores the message about not releasing fats and releases triglycerides (stored fats) into your bloodstream. These triglycerides are contained in VLDLs (very low density lipoproteins), which are usually rendered harmless by enzymes in your blood. But the enzymes at that moment are dealing with the fat from your food so the VLDLs can end up forming plaque on your artery walls.

In 2009, the American Heart Association published a scientific statement in their journal *Circulation* entitled *Dietary sugar intake and cardiovascular health*[15], in which they expressed concern that sugar and refined carbohydrates can increase triglycerides (a known risk factor for heart disease), while lowering levels of HDL. HDL is the 'good' cholesterol which would normally remove cholesterol from the arteries (LDL is the 'bad' cholesterol). If HDL is low, cholesterol could build up in the blood vessels. They also pointed out that high sugar consumption is associated with an increase in inflammation and oxidative stress, both of which increase the risk of heart problems.

When your body produces the stress hormones adrenaline and cortisol, in response to blood sugar swings, the effect of cortisol in your body is to cause inflammation. However, the inflammation stops your body using insulin efficiently, so it tries to compensate by making yet more insulin, which in turn causes more inflammation and leaves you stuck in a vicious cycle.

It is now thought that inflammation is the key factor not only in heart disease but also in most of our degenerative illnesses, such as type 2 diabetes and Alzheimer's. You will see this connection made clearer and clearer throughout this book. As cholesterol travels around your arteries it will only start to form plaque if your blood vessels are inflamed. Inflammation damages the lining of the arteries, making it easy for the fatty plaque to stick. Over time, this fatty deposit can break away from the blood vessel and cause either a heart attack or stroke, depending on whether it blocks the blood supply to your heart or your brain.

It is possible to measure how much inflammation is present in your body by measuring a marker called C-reactive protein through a blood test.

Another useful marker is homocysteine: If this is high in your blood, it is not only linked to increased inflammation but also to an increased risk of clots and thickening of the artery walls. Homocysteine is an amino acid which is naturally produced in your body; it breaks down another amino acid called methionine. Homocysteine should be successfully detoxified and excreted by your body but if this does not happen it can increase inflammation. The B vitamins (in particular B6, B12 and folic acid) control this detoxification so if you have deficiencies in these vitamins, you can end up with high levels of homocysteine.

Research has shown that taking B vitamins in supplement form not only reduced homocysteine levels but also improved the health of the blood vessels[16]. For a simple finger prick homocysteine test go to www.naturalhealthpractice.com.

The statins connection

Another interesting connection between cholesterol and blood sugar is that if you take statins to lower cholesterol you are actually increasing your risk of type 2 diabetes, possibly by up to 46 per cent[17]. The higher the dose of the statins, the higher the risk. Research also shows that people with genetically high cholesterol are less likely to have type 2 diabetes[18].

There does not seem to be agreement on why lowering cholesterol would increase the risk of diabetes. A theory has been proposed that statins activate a specific inflammatory immune response, which stops insulin being effective. So the suggestion is that people who are on statins should take a drug used to treat diabetes, called glyburide, to offset the risk[19].

I often see patients come to my clinic who are on numerous drugs, many of them being taken purely to offset the side effects of the others. That is exactly what is being suggested here with statins and glyburide. Statins increase the risk of diabetes so, instead of treating the problem of high cholesterol (which I don't think is a major problem anyway), people are told to take another drug, a diabetes drug, to overcome the side effect.

But glyburide carries its own side effects. The most common are heartburn and nausea so then the person may be prescribed antacids or proton pump inhibitors (PPIs) to stop these side effects. But the PPIs increase the risk of osteoporosis which will, in turn, need medication and so it goes on.

Maybe it has nothing to do with the statins and maybe it is reducing cholesterol that increases the risk of diabetes. Because we know, as mentioned above, that people with genetically high cholesterol (who are not on statins) have a lower risk of diabetes.

We also know that if cholesterol is lowered too much it can increase the risk of depression and suicidal tendencies. The brain needs a certain amount of cholesterol to release brain neurotransmitters and, if cholesterol goes lower than 4 mmol/L, people are more likely to die from cancer, liver disease and strokes[20].

As well as the risks of increasing diabetes and cancer if cholesterol is reduced too low, there are other possible side effects from statins; digestive problems, nausea, headaches and sleep disturbances. They are also known to cause muscle pain, night cramps, memory loss and sexual problems.

For women taking statins who already have heart disease, this medication has not been shown to increase life expectancy[21] but has been shown to increase the risk of breast cancer[22].

There has been some interesting research on the whole issue of cholesterol and heart disease. In one study over 130,000 patients admitted to hospital with a heart attack were tested for cholesterol levels and it was found they had lower levels of cholesterol than normal, not higher[23]. Even when the researchers looked at levels of the supposedly 'bad' LDL cholesterol, the people with the lowest LDL levels had twice the death rate three years later[24].

The key may lie in having optimum levels of the 'good' HDL cholesterol. It seems that having too much sugar in your blood 'kills' HDL. There is a substance called methylglyoxal (MG) formed by the sugar in your blood which alters the structure of HDL and makes it less effective. HDL is 'good' because it removes excess levels of bad cholesterol from your body. Higher levels of MG have been found in people with diabetes[25].

Only 20 per cent of the cholesterol in your bloodstream comes from what you eat; the remaining 80 per cent is produced by your liver. Statins work by blocking the production of the cholesterol from your liver. The question must always be, why is your liver producing too much cholesterol? This brings us back to the vital connection between your liver and blood sugar balance. It is the message insulin sends out that causes your liver to produce too much cholesterol in general and too much 'bad' LDL cholesterol in particular. Get your blood sugar back in balance and you will not only allow your lipid levels to settle back into the normal range but you will also be reducing inflammation.

I've mentioned the connection of sugar to type 2 diabetes already but in the next chapter we'll look more closely at this growing problem in our health.

CHAPTER 6

Sugar and Type 2 Diabetes

The UK has the fastest growing rate of diabetes in the developed world, with 2.7 million people suffering from it, a colossal rise of 450 per cent from 1960. Nearly one million more people are estimated to have type 2 diabetes and don't even know it. We also have children as young as nine and ten in the UK with type 2 diabetes, which previously was known as late onset or middle aged diabetes.

The toll of type 2 diabetes is costing the NHS £9 billion a year and, shockingly, results in 7,000 lower leg amputations a year.

But this is also a world-wide problem. In Mexico, in 2006, they realised that diabetes, the country's leading cause of death, had doubled since 2000 and, with 75,000 amputations a year caused by diabetes and a major obesity crisis not only in adults but also in children (between 1999 and 2006 obesity rose by 40 per cent in children aged 5-11), they decided to put a ten per cent tax on soft drinks in 2014. This has resulted in a ten per cent decrease in soft drink consumption and a revenue of 1.9 billion pesos. It could be argued that if they collected so much revenue then people did not stop buying soft drinks, they just paid more for them. But, in 2014, the sales of taxed drinks fell by six per cent and sales of bottle water were up by four per cent.

China also now has a major public health crisis caused by type 2 diabetes with more than 100 million affected by the disease. This crisis has an annual projected cost of 360 billion yuan (approx. £36 billion). It is thought that the increase in type 2 diabetes has been driven by the introduction of a more Westernised diet, resulting in an increase in rates of obesity, together with a reduction in physical activity and psychosocial stress[26].

Doctors also use a diagnosis of 'prediabetes' and recent research has shown that one in three adults (35.3 per cent) in the UK has prediabetes, compared to 11.6 per cent in 2003[27]. It's an enormous, and worrying, rise. In China, latest estimates indicate that around half of Chinese adults have prediabetes, putting them at high risk of developing type 2 diabetes and multiple related illnesses.

A diagnosis of prediabetes is given when someone's blood glucose levels are higher than normal but not quite into the type 2 diabetic range. If that person does not make changes in their diet and lifestyle, they are highly likely to become a type 2 diabetic, usually within five years of the initial diagnosis.

It seems logical that a problem with blood sugar would be linked to the sugar that we eat, but for many years this concept has been dismissed. Experts have been quite adamant that sugar does not cause diabetes, instead blaming the fat we eat. The argument went that, because 'fat was fattening', it was an increase in overweight people that was causing the rise in diabetes. Yes, being overweight *does* increase the risk of diabetes but the weight gain comes from sugary foods *not* the fats. There is a huge amount of ignorance around sugar, even in medical and academic circles. As an amusing aside, I have even been at an academic conference where one speaker was adamant that sugar did not cause tooth decay!

How insulin controls blood sugar

Let's have a look at how insulin controls your blood sugar. As we've already seen, insulin is a hormone produced by your pancreas whose role is to help move glucose (sugar) after a meal out of your blood and into your muscles to give you energy.

You have insulin receptors on your cells that act like a lock and key system. The receptors are the lock and insulin is the key. Insulin opens the lock and glucose (sugar) from your bloodstream is able to move into your cells. This means that your cells can use the glucose for energy and, at the same time, the amount of glucose in your blood is lowered because it has been moved out of your bloodstream.

However, if you live on a roller coaster of highs and lows of blood sugar swings you can, over a period of time, become insulin resistant. The insulin receptors do not open in response to insulin and the glucose from your blood is not moved into your cells. This means you are not getting the energy you need from your food and also that you end up with high blood glucose (sugar).

Symptoms of prediabetes

There are not many clear-cut symptoms relating to prediabetes. However, you might see darkened skin on certain areas of your body - a condition known as acanthosis nigricans. This is often found between your elbow and shoulder and, at first, you might think your skin is just dirty. You can also develop skin tags (acrohorda), floppy bits of skin that can grow anywhere but are most commonly found on the neck, underarms and eyelids. Skin tags don't necessarily indicate prediabetes but they can show that your blood sugar is not as balanced as it should be.

Regardless of any symptoms, it is suggested that you are checked for prediabetes if you are:

- Overweight with a BMI of over 25.
- Over the age of 45.

Plus you have any of these other risk factors:

- Strong family history risk of type 2 diabetes.
- Physically inactive.
- History of gestational diabetes or giving birth to a baby weighing more than nine pounds.
- Have/had PCOS (polycystic ovary syndrome).
- Have high triglycerides or low 'good' HDL cholesterol.

Symptoms of type 2 diabetes

You should see your doctor to be tested for type 2 diabetes if you have any of the following symptoms:

- Increased thirst.
- Frequent urination.
- Fatigue.
- Blurred vision.

Links with food manufacturers

As already mentioned, it is going to be a long hard battle to change public perceptions about fat and sugar, and which is the culprit behind most of our major illnesses. As we've already seen, a major problem is that many of the organisations that advise people on their food choices have links to food manufacturers and it is going to be difficult, probably impossible, to say that certain foods are unhealthy if the companies that manufacture those foods are supplying the organisations with funding. It would be like biting the hand that feeds.

The American Academy of Nutrition and Dietetics (formerly the American Dietetic Association) has been shown to receive funding from food companies such as Coca Cola, McDonald's, PepsiCo, Mars, Kellogg's, Hershey and The Sugar Association. They say that: 'It's important for ADA to be at the same table with food companies because of the positive influence that we can have on them. For ADA, relationships with outside organizations are not about promoting companies' products; they are about creating nutrition messages that people can understand and act upon to improve their health and that of their families'[28].

The benefits lie firmly with the food companies as it looks as though they are working with health professionals and dieticians in making their foods healthier. It's a short leap in the public imagination to consider that they have an 'endorsement' from nutritional organisations.

The British Dietetic Association has alliances with a number of different companies, one of which is a breakfast bar containing sugar and also a probiotic drink containing sugar (www.bda.uk.com/about/workwithus/currentcorpmembers).

What is the difference between the different types of diabetes?

All types of diabetes involve higher than normal levels of sugar (glucose) in the blood but the causes are different.

Type 1 diabetes is often diagnosed in childhood (although some people can be diagnosed later in life). It is classed as an auto-immune problem because the person's own immune system kills the cells (beta-cells) in the pancreas that produce insulin. This means that a type 1 diabetic needs to have insulin injections (or an insulin pump) for the rest of his or her life in order to survive.

Type 2 diabetes is often called middle-aged onset diabetes, because it develops later in life and is often associated with being overweight. In type 2 diabetes, the pancreas does produce insulin but the body stops responding to it and the person becomes insulin resistant. So the pancreas will try to produce more insulin to overcome this resistance. The first line of treatment in type 2 diabetes is insulin sensitising medication. But if the pancreas keeps having to overwork then the beta cells in the pancreas may fail and insulin injections or a pump will be required.

Type 3 diabetes? A new diagnosis of type 3 diabetes has been suggested for Alzheimer's disease. Research has shown that insulin resistance can cause Alzheimer's disease to develop[29]. It has also been shown that treatment with insulin sensitisers used in cases of type 2 diabetes can improve brain function and also slow the rate of cognitive decline in Alzheimer's. The same researchers have said that many type 2 diabetics have deposits of protein (amyloid beta) in their pancreas which is similar to that found in the brain with Alzheimer's.

It is already known that people with type 2 diabetes have an increased risk of developing Alzheimer's (about 50-65 per cent higher). It may be possible to work on both prevention and the slowing down of the progression of both diseases in the same way, as the cause is effectively the same.

It has been shown that high sugar is a predictor of type 2 diabetes, regardless of someone's weight. Research from Stanford University 'provides the first large-scale, population-based evidence for the idea that not all calories are equal from a diabetes risk standpoint' and that sugar has 'a direct, independent link to diabetes'[30].

The research showed that for every 150 calories (from sugar) consumed above the recommended daily calorie intake there was an eleven-fold increase in the rate of type 2 diabetes, compared to when the 150 extra calories came from non-sugar foods or drink.

A European study has also shown that having just one sugar-sweetened drink a day increases the risk of type 2 diabetes by 22 per cent[31]. This is interesting research because much of the information about sugar-sweetened drinks has come from America, where there are clear links between sugary drinks and diabetes. It is helpful to know that this applies just as much to Europe as it does to America. The other interesting part of this research is that pure fruit juice does not increase the risk of diabetes.

However, if you substitute artificially-sweetened drinks for sugar-sweetened ones, the risks remain. They also increase your risk of type 2 diabetes. Research from France, tracking over 66,000 women over 14 years, found that the risk of developing type 2 diabetes was higher for women who drank either artificially-sweetened or sugar-sweetened drinks. However, the really interesting part was that the risk was even higher for those who drank the artificially-sweetened ones, compared to the sugar-sweetened ones. Half a litre of artificially sweetened drinks increased the risk by 15 per cent but 1.5 litres caused a 59 per cent higher risk. This study once again showed there was no link between drinking 100 per cent fruit juices and risk of diabetes[32].

Testing for type 2 diabetes

For many years, a blood test looking at fasting glucose has been the major way of diagnosing diabetes. Why fasting? Because having any food before the test would automatically cause glucose to rise in response to the food and give a false reading. It was important to know how high the glucose levels were without food triggering the response.

If there was any doubt over the diagnosis then an oral glucose tolerance test was performed. Again this required the person to fast overnight and in the morning he or she would be given a drink containing glucose. A blood sample was then taken two hours later. In a non-diabetic person, the level of glucose would not be too high. But a high level over 11.1mmol/L would indicate diabetes.

Once diagnosed with diabetes then a test called HbA1c (glycosylated haemoglobin) would have been performed every few months - this gives an indication of the average blood glucose over the previous two to three months.

It has now been recommended that the HbA1c test should be used instead of fasting glucose to diagnose diabetes, as it seems to be more accurate at identifying those at risk. An HbA1c level of 48 mmol/mol (6.5 per cent) or more is considered a diagnosis of diabetes.

HbA1c, glycosylated haemoglobin, is a measure of how much glucose is attached to part of the red blood cells (the haemoglobin). It measures the amount of glycation that has affected the haemoglobin. I discuss glycation in more detail in the chapter on sugar and ageing. The problem with glycation is that it causes free radical damage, which is linked to premature ageing, heart disease and cancer.

As we have already seen, there is a step before full-blown diabetes known as prediabetes or borderline diabetes. If a person with prediabetes doesn't take action in changing his or her diet or lifestyle then it will progress into type 2 diabetes. A diagnosis of prediabetes would be given if the HbA1c level is 42-47 mmol/mol (6-6.4 per cent).

I remember a lovely lady coming to see me in the clinic who had been given a diagnosis of prediabetes and told by her doctor to 'come back when she was diabetic'! She had come to me because she didn't want to become diabetic and knew that she was at a stage where her health could go one of two ways. Either it would progress to type 2 diabetes so she would be on medication for life, or else she could reverse the prognosis by changing her diet and looking at her lifestyle. She was very keen to reverse it. How many people just accept that full-blown diabetes is inevitable? It's not.

This measurement of HbA1c has much larger implications than only indicating the risk of diabetes. It is well known that people with diabetes are at increased risk of developing certain cancers, compared to non-diabetics; including womb, liver, pancreatic, kidney, oesophageal, bowel, breast and bladder cancer[33].

New research has looked at whether the level of HbA1c can be used as a predictor for cancer development, independent of diabetes[34]. One study concluded that 'the incidence of cancer in the diabetic and non-diabetic populations could, therefore, potentially be reduced by decreasing glucose levels. This could be achieved by means of appropriate lifestyle or therapeutic interventions, and by imposing stricter recommendations for glycaemic control.'

If you would like to find out your level of HbA1c then do get in touch as it can be organised at one of my clinics. See the *Resources* section at the back of this book.

Testing for insulin resistance

There is a more comprehensive blood test which not only measures HbA1c but also other factors that are connected under the term 'metabolic syndrome'. This blood test measures HbA1c plus insulin; cholesterol including HDL ('good'), LDL ('bad'), VLDL (very low density lipoprotein - 'very bad'); the ratio of total cholesterol to HDL cholesterol; triglycerides and the ratio of triglycerides to HDL cholesterol; plus high sensitive C-reactive protein (a marker of inflammation).

This is a fasting blood test, which means that you have the blood taken first thing in the morning without eating or drinking. A kit would be sent to you which you can then take to your local practice nurse or doctor so they can take a small quantity of blood. This is sent to the laboratory and the results are forwarded onto you with an explanation.

For more information on this test which can be organised by post see the *Resources* section.

I cannot stress how important it is to bring your blood sugar under control; not only to prevent type 2 diabetes but also to prevent cancer and for other aspects of your health which we will discuss in the following chapters. The effect of sugar has such a far-reaching effect on your health that it is hard to see why this information has not been made more widespread. Let's redress the balance. Armed with the right information, you can make informed choices and radically improve your present health and future-protect your body as well.

In the next chapter we will turn to the connections between a diet high in sugar and Alzheimer's and dementia.

CHAPTER 7

Sugar and Alzheimer's/Dementia

As we have seen in the last chapter, it has now been suggested that Alzheimer's is, effectively, 'diabetes' of the brain. Some researchers claim that the two illnesses are so similar that Alzheimer's should really be called 'type 3 diabetes'. This could explain why almost three quarters of people suffering from type 2 diabetes go on to develop Alzheimer's: A staggering 70 per cent of people with this form of diabetes go on to develop Alzheimer's, compared to only ten per cent of people without diabetes.

Research on rats fed to develop type 2 diabetes showed that the animals' concentration deteriorated rapidly as the disease progressed[35]. The high levels of insulin blocked a group of enzymes which break down amyloid. Amyloid is an abnormal protein, usually produced in your bone marrow, which can be deposited in any tissue or organ. The amyloid builds up into toxic clumps (plaque) which disrupts neurological function.

What is the difference between Alzheimer's and dementia?

Brain function does change as we become older. The symptoms that are associated with a gradual decline in brain function, for example loss of memory and difficulty in concentrating, are described as dementia. The two main forms of dementia are Alzheimer's (the most common) and vascular dementia. Alzheimer's is caused by plaque (beta amyloid plaque) and tangles developing in the brain. Plaques are clumpy spheres that float between the neurons and prevent the transmission of messages to each other; the tangles actually choke the neurons from inside. Vascular dementia is a problem with the supply of blood to the brain.

The risks of dementia increase with age and affect about five per cent of people over the age of 65. Dementia is much more common in women and is now the biggest killer for women, causing three times more deaths than breast cancer.

Not all insulin is produced by your pancreas

It has now been shown that it's not just your pancreas that produces insulin; your brain has its own supply. Your brain needs insulin for the survival of brain cells. A low level of insulin in the brain is linked to degeneration of brain cells; conversely, good levels of insulin are essential for survival of brain cells.

Research looking at postmortem brain tissue of people with Alzheimer's has shown that insulin levels were reduced in the frontal cortex, hippocampus and hypothalamus, all the areas that are affected by the disease[36]. But the cerebellum, which is not affected by Alzheimer's, did not show the same low level of insulin.

Beta amyloid is a protein in the brain and, when healthy, has certain functions such as an immune function (fighting microbes), transporting cholesterol and protecting against oxidative stress. It is interesting to see that beta amyloid is connected with cholesterol as I've already explained. It only becomes a problem when it forms clumps (plaque) and this was first noted by Alois Alzheimer after whom the disease is named.

Obviously, the most important question is why does beta amyloid start forming clumps and tangles? Finding the trigger would undoubtedly help in the prevention of Alzheimer's. It is thought that the cause might lie with insulin and how it functions in the brain.

Up until a few years ago, it was thought that insulin simply regulated blood sugar but it is now understood that it has a number of other functions as well. It regulates neurotransmitters, brain chemicals like acetylcholine, which are important for learning and memory. It is important for healthy neuron function, especially in those areas of the brain most affected by Alzheimer's - the hippocampus and the frontal lobe.

Insulin is also important for the growth of blood vessels which help supply the brain with oxygen and glucose (you will see the relevance of this when we look at cancer). This role is important for vascular dementia when the blood supply to the brain is restricted. Insulin is also important for promoting plasticity, whereby your brain can change over your lifetime, making new connections. It was previously thought that our brains were fixed but we now know that change within the brain is constant, with some connections being strengthened and others being weakened.

This effect of insulin has been confirmed in animals; if they are made to become diabetic, Alzheimer's changes in the brain occur with an increase in the beta amyloid plaque[37].

The suggestion is that, like the body, the brain can become insulin resistant, unable to respond to insulin properly. This has been demonstrated in the brains of human corpses. Researchers took brain cells from people who had been diagnosed with Alzheimer's, and those who hadn't, and soaked them in insulin (brain signalling is maintained for a number of hours after death).

The brain tissue from those without Alzheimer's showed active insulin signalling in response to the insulin but in those with Alzheimer's there was no such activity, particularly in the hippocampus which is the centre for learning and cognitive function. The conclusion was that people with Alzheimer's have brain insulin resistance[38].

I cannot stress enough how important it is that you follow the recommendations in this book and eliminate (or, at the very least, drastically reduce) added sugar and also refined carbohydrates (like white bread and white pasta) from your diet. You don't even have to have prediabetes or full blown type 2 diabetes for these negative brain changes to start taking effect.

In one study, people were either given a high glycaemic index (GI) diet or a low GI diet. Within just four weeks, those on the high GI diet had higher levels of insulin and significantly higher levels of beta amyloid taken from spinal fluid, compared to those on the low GI diet[39].

Just having higher levels of glucose from eating too much sugary food is a risk factor for dementia even if you don't have diabetes[40].

It is also thought that inflammation plays a key role in Alzheimer's and dementia. It may change blood flow in the brain in the same way that it does for the blood supply to the heart, as I've already described. It is also thought that, in cases of Alzheimer's, inflammation worsens the beta amyloid inflamed areas and literally ages the neurons, hence speeding up the usual age-related decline.

Being on this blood sugar roller coaster not only causes issues with glucose and insulin (which in themselves will increase the risk of Alzheimer's) but it will also cause the release of cortisol. Cortisol, over time, will cause an increase in inflammation which, in turn, will worsen brain and memory function much more swiftly.

Another way of thinking about cortisol is as the direct opposite to melatonin. Both these hormones have a circadian rhythm - they are at different levels at various parts of the day and night. Cortisol is higher in the morning, revving us up ready to start the day, and then reduces at night. Melatonin is higher at night and then decreases by the morning. However, if the cortisol level stays high, then the melatonin level will be low.

It has been noticed that people with Alzheimer's exhibit an effect called 'sundowning' when their symptoms follow a circadian rhythm and get worse towards the end of the day[41]. Production of beta amyloid also follows a circadian rhythm that increases during the day and reduces when the person sleeps. But if mice are deprived of sleep then there is an increase in beta amyloid of 25 per cent[42].

So the sleep/wake cycle may have a part to play in Alzheimer's. The suggestion is that it could be connected to melatonin but it is just as likely that it is associated with cortisol, as this hormone is definitely related to the blood sugar roller coaster.

Get your blood sugar in balance by reducing and eliminating hidden sugar from your foods. Make sure you are getting enough sleep and good quality sleep. We know that light exposure, especially the 'blue' light from phones and TV can reduce melatonin and many people will use laptops and phones in bed just before going to sleep.

In the next chapter we'll move on to look at how sugar can play a part in cancer.

CHAPTER 8

Sugar and Cancer

We know that insulin is a 'grower'. As we've seen, it can make skin tags grow on your neck and armpits and, unfortunately, it can have the same effect on tumours inside your body.

High levels of insulin have been linked to cancers of the bowel, liver, pancreas, ovary and womb[43]. We have already seen that insulin is important for the growth of blood vessels. This can be a good thing in the brain, where we want a healthy supply of oxygen. However, a process called angiogenesis, in which new blood vessels are formed, is a mechanism which keeps tumours growing because it provides them with a blood supply.

Angiogenesis is a normal process that helps with growth and wound healing, but it also has this negative effect with regard to tumours and is one of the mechanisms which helps turn a benign tumour into a malignant (cancerous) one.

Sugar feeds cancer

As far back as the 1950s, a scientist called Otto Warburg discovered that cancer cells have a different form of energy metabolism in comparison to healthy cells[44].

Cancer cells function in a different way to healthy cells showing an increase in a process called 'anaerobic glycolysis'. This means that they use glucose (sugar) as their primary fuel. So if your blood glucose levels are high, there will inevitably be excess glucose on which the cancer cells can 'feed'. There's no doubt about it: Sugar is fuel for cancer cells.

In addition, cortisol, which is released in higher amounts in response to the blood sugar roller coaster, reduces the number of cells called 'natural killer cells'. These normally work to help your immune system identify cancer cells as well as viruses. Cortisol also encourages new blood vessels to form to tumours (angiogenesis) which can stimulate their growth.

This effect of glucose was studied in a trial with over 49,000 postmenopausal women. The researchers found that women with a high carbohydrate and sugar intake had a significantly higher risk of breast cancer. Postmenopausal women who ate foods with a high glycaemic index (sugar, white flour, convenience foods) were 87 per cent more likely to develop breast cancer than those on healthier, low GI diets. The risk was particularly strong for women who had used HRT or who did no physical exercise[45].

Even just having higher blood sugar levels significantly increases your risk of getting and dying of cancer, regardless of whether you are overweight or not. This is according to research on over 500,000 men and women with an average age of 44. The bad news is that the connection with blood sugar and cancer is even stronger for women and for fatal cancers[46].

Having higher levels of insulin can give you a threefold increased risk of breast cancer. Over 5,400 women were divided into three groups, depending on their insulin levels, and followed over eight years. Those women in the group with the highest levels of insulin had the largest risk of breast cancer and this was again independent of their weight. Being overweight does increase the risk of breast cancer but these results showed that blood sugar and insulin are the major risk factors[47].

Insulin is classed as an anabolic steroid (a 'grower or builder' of cells) and one of the things it does is to encourage cells to mutate. It also stops a process called apoptosis; literally cell suicide. Healthy cells are normally programmed to die when they have fulfilled their function. If apoptosis is not happening then uncontrolled cell division can take place, as it does in cancer.

New test for cancer

Using an MRI scanner, scientists have been able to identify cancer by tracking how sugar is absorbed in the body. We know that malignant tumours consume much more sugar (glucose), up to ten to twelve times the rate of healthy tissue, in order to feed their rapid growth. Tumours glowed when using the same sugar content found in half a standard sized chocolate bar[48].

All of this information is important for preventing cancer, because by eliminating or reducing your added sugar intake you are literally starving cancer cells of their fuel. It is equally as important if you have already had cancer and are working on preventing a recurrence. Research has shown that bringing blood sugar under control should be part of cancer therapy, as high sugar intake is associated with poor survival rates after diagnosis of early breast cancer.

When HbA1c, glycosylated haemoglobin (a measure of glucose level) was measured in a group of cancer patients (some with active disease and some in remission), the scientists found a statistically-significant lower average blood glucose in those in remission[49].

Once again, the message is clear. Do your body a favour and cut sugar out of your life - before it cuts your life short.

In the next chapter we will look at how sugar affects the stress response. Is sugar the reason you often feel irritable, angry, depressed or forgetful? It's quite possible.

CHAPTER 9

Sugar and Stress

Do any of these symptoms sound familiar? Run through the following checklist and tick off the ones that you experience on a regular basis:

- Irritability.
- Aggressive outbursts.
- Nervousness, fear and anxiety.
- Depression.
- Crying spells.
- Dizziness.
- Confusion, forgetfulness, inability to concentrate.
- Fatigue.
- Insomnia.
- Headaches.
- Palpitations.
- Muscle cramps.
- Excess sweating.
- Digestive problems.
- Allergies.
- Lack of sex drive.

These are all symptoms of low blood sugar also known as hypoglycaemia. When your blood sugar rises too high, more insulin has to be released to deal with the high blood sugar which then, in turn, causes your body to crash into hypoglycaemia. Firstly, it sends you off for that quick fix of a cup of tea and biscuit or a bar of chocolate. Secondly, it releases your stress hormones adrenaline and cortisol. Cortisol is the hormone that gives the message to your liver to release your stores of glucose (sugar). With both these actions, your body is trying to lift your low blood sugar level.

You can see that it would be useful for your sugar stores to be released when your stress hormones are produced in a genuine survival situation where you are going to need instant energy to run or fight for your life. But, in this situation, your stress hormones are being released just because of the way you are eating.

The stress hormones will also cause you to have higher glucose levels because they automatically lower insulin when they are released. As we've already seen, this was really useful in evolutionary terms because when we were running away from a wild animal, for instance, we would need as much glucose as possible in our bloodstream to give us extra energy.

But, in everyday life nowadays, we are not running away from wild animals and our stress is pretty constant: most people live with chronic stress. But the impact on our bodies and the amount of stress we feel is made worse by eating sugary foods, which cause the release of the stress hormones.

As more and more cortisol is released, more glucose is produced which causes high blood glucose levels. Insulin levels are dampened in order to keep high blood glucose which, essentially, makes the cells insulin resistant. With chronic stress, cortisol is sending the same message out all the time. The pancreas desperately tries to produce more insulin; blood glucose will stay high but the glucose can't get into the cells and so it goes on, in a vicious cycle.

It is well known that stress can make it difficult for a person with type 2 diabetes to control their blood sugar levels. Severe stress can cause insulin resistance even in people without diabetes. It can also change how the pancreas functions[50].

To make the vicious cycle even worse, stress changes how you eat and the choices you make. Stress makes you reach for those comforting sugary foods. Because stress hormones were released, your body thinks you have either run or fought for your life, so it believes it needs to refuel and restock, just in case there is going to be another life-threatening event coming around the corner. Hence, it will increase your appetite to hoard calories because the next stress may be a famine – so it will send you off for those quick fixes to restock your energy stores quickly[51].

Our food selection definitely changes under stress. Interestingly, it seems to affect women more than men, with women often not just eating more food in general but also choosing those foods that they would avoid under normal circumstances as they know they are unhealthy. Research shows that people are eating these foods in order to feel better. However, I also think it has an evolutionary benefit reaching back to when we led lives that were fraught with jeopardy most of the time, with the frequent threat of famine as well as the danger of wild animals[52].

Controlling stress

You can't ever totally avoid stress. Nowadays, stress is triggered by a huge range of psychological factors and external events. We become stressed by relationships, by work, by finances, even by social interactions and how we perceive ourselves on social media. Obviously, some of these can be controlled by looking within ourselves but not everything in modern life can be controlled.

However, you can definitely control your blood sugar roller coaster. That in itself will reduce the amount of stress hormones that are being released and you will automatically feel calmer in yourself.

Stress test

There is a simple test you can take to find out how stressed you are. It is not possible to measure adrenaline because it is so fast-acting. However, that is not a problem as we can look at cortisol - the effects of cortisol remain in your body for a long time. The test is simple, safe and non-invasive - it can determine both your cortisol and DHEA levels using four saliva samples. These can easily be collected at home or at work and sent off in the post.

DHEA (dehydroepiandrosterone), which is another hormone produced by your adrenal glands, works to balance many of the negative effects of cortisol on your body, helping it cope with stress. In research studies, DHEA has been shown to improve memory function and boost energy levels[53].

Balance is the key in assessing the overall effect of the adrenal hormones in your body. If these two hormones, cortisol and DHEA, become chronically 'out of sync', it can tax your body's immune system, making you less able to cope with stress and more susceptible to a wide range of illnesses.

After analysing your results, you will be sent a report showing how your adrenal glands are functioning and if there are any imbalances that need to be corrected. See www.naturalhealthpractice.com for information and to organise an Adrenal Stress Test.

Cortisol levels rise dramatically with stress, prolonging your body's 'fight or flight' response. If your body is producing too much or too little cortisol, you may feel some of the following symptoms.

- **Weakness and fatigue**
Cortisol imbalances can throw off the body's blood sugar metabolism, making you feel weak, tired and run-down. Too much cortisol can also interfere with sleep patterns and produce a 'wakeful' unrelaxing sleep state. So you may feel worn-out even after a full night's sleep.

- **Muscle and joint pain**

Excess cortisol in the bloodstream accelerates the breakdown of body tissue and prevents proper tissue repair, leading to muscle and joint injuries and chronic pain.

- **Obesity**

Cortisol imbalances can stimulate fat deposits in various parts of the body, resulting in weight gains in the trunk, chest, neck, and face.

- **Poor skin**

High levels of cortisol can reduce the skin's ability to regenerate, resulting in an unhealthy skin appearance.

Over time, cortisol imbalances can take a heavy toll on your health, wearing down your immune system, triggering premature ageing and setting the stage for chronic illness. Anxiety, depression, heart disease and osteoporosis have all been linked with elevated cortisol levels.

Are you stressed?

Do you find it difficult to get up in the mornings? Have your periods stopped or become irregular? Are you constantly under pressure and/or overloaded? A wide range of physical and emotional disorders have been linked to stress which, in turn, can relate to adrenal hormone imbalances.

Ask yourself the following questions:

- Do you often feel weak and tired, for no apparent reason?
- Are you under chronic stress?
- Do you have trouble getting a night of restful sleep?
- Do you have low sex drive?
- Are you exposed to high noise levels?
- Are you feeling anxious or depressed?
- Do you have menstrual difficulties?
- Are you suffering from joint pain?
- Do you have an eating disorder?
- Have you recently gained or lost weight?
- Do you suffer from ulcers or irritable bowel syndrome?
- Do you have trouble with concentration, memory or learning?
- Do you suffer from hypertension?

If you answered yes to any of these questions, you may be suffering from an over- or under-reactive stress response by your adrenal hormones.

Another interesting connection with cholesterol is that DHEA is produced from cholesterol, so if you have low cholesterol levels then you may not be able to produce enough DHEA. DHEA opposes cortisol so the lower the DHEA, the stronger the effects of this stress hormone.

So sugar and stress are inextricably linked. As we will see in the next chapter, sugar is also the reason why many of us age prematurely.

CHAPTER 10

Sugar and Ageing

Still not persuaded that you need to give up sugar? If all the other information about sugar's health risks have not been enough to persuade you to make some changes in what you eat, then how about the fact that sugar makes you age more swiftly? This accelerated ageing process can be seen on the outside, not just on the inside.

A few years back, scientists from the Leiden University Medical Centre in the Netherlands measured the blood levels of 600 men and women aged between 50 and 70. They then showed photographs of these men and women to independent people and found that those with the highest blood sugar (glucose) levels looked older than the ones with the lowest levels. They found that for every 1mm/l increase in blood sugar, people thought that person looked five months older[54]. The scientists had controlled for other factors, such as smoking, yet the fact remains the higher the blood sugar the older the person appeared.

Sugar makes your skin lose its elasticity and plumpness. This is all down to a process called glycation. Glycation is the bonding between sugar and protein in the body, making proteins like collagen and elastin become less effective. This glycation effect results in the formation of highly toxic chemicals called 'advanced glycation end-products' (AGEs). These AGEs become deposited in the dermal matrix of the skin, causing the skin to harden and lose its elasticity[55].

Collagen helps to plump out your skin, giving it a soft, younger look. Elastin gives your skin elasticity so that when you smile or frown your skin can withdraw back to its original place.

AGEs make both collagen and elastin become rigid, stiff and inflexible so wrinkles form, skin can become discoloured (brown spots can form, often known as 'liver spots') and skin generally becomes dry, dull and fragile. While that hardening is going on in the skin, the same thing is happening in your body with hardened arteries and stiff joints. Glycation is why diabetics can age prematurely and why they often have artery, kidney and nerve damage.

I mentioned earlier that nowadays, when you are tested for blood glucose levels, it is recommended that HbAlc, glycosylated haemoglobin, is measured instead of fasting glucose. This measures the amount of glycation that has affected the haemoglobin. Glycation is just as damaging inside where it can't be seen as on the outside, where it is clearly visible in the form of wrinkles.

Telomeres

As well as AGEs, another way we age is connected to DNA structures called telomeres. These are the protective caps at the end of your chromosomes – rather like the hard ends on shoelaces. Telomeres become shorter as we get older and the quicker they shorten, the faster we age. Inflammation causes telomeres to shorten and we know that sugar causes an inflammatory reaction in the body[56].

This shortening of the telomeres connected to sugar intake has been studied on more than 5,000 people. Researchers found that those who drank the most sugary soft drinks had shorter telomeres. The shorter the telomere, the harder it is for a cell to regenerate and so your body gets older faster. The researchers found that just two cans of soft drink (20 US fl. oz. or 600ml) are linked to an additional 4.6 years of ageing – similar to the effect of smoking. Interestingly, they found that drinking 100 per cent fruit juice was marginally associated with longer telomeres[57].

I think the message is clear: if you want to slow down the ageing process, you need to do it from the inside out. By cutting out sugar, you not only prevent or lessen the risk of many of our degenerative illnesses like cancer, heart disease and type 2 diabetes, but you also slow down the signs of ageing from the outside, reducing the visible signs of wrinkles, and hard and discoloured skin.

I'm aware that the last few chapters haven't made for cheerful reading. However, I feel it's essential you realise just how bad sugar really is; what terrible damage it does to your health, your wellbeing, your mood and even your looks.

In the next chapter, we will start to look at what you can do to prevent the ill-effects of sugar. Even if you've been over-consuming sugar for years, it's not too late. Let's look at how to make changes; exciting changes.

CHAPTER 11

What are the Alternatives?

I hope I have made a conclusive case for cutting out sugar. Where possible, it is always better to rely on the natural sweetness of foods themselves rather than on using sugar or artificial sweeteners. However, I do recognise that there are times when you may want to add some extra sweetness to a food.

Sometimes there are easy shifts you can make.

If you are making cakes, think of ways other than sugar to add sweetness. For example, you could add carrots, raisins, dates, figs or bananas as natural sweeteners. Many people now make wonderful cakes from naturally sweet vegetables such as beetroot and carrot. For apple pies or crumbles, use eating apples instead of cooking apples so you do not need to add sugar – you could always add raisins or sultanas to make a pie or crumble that little bit sweeter. Unsweetened date slice is wonderful because dates are naturally sweet. Some spices like cinnamon and vanilla also add sweetness and flavour, enabling you to reduce the amount of other sweeteners in a recipe or remove them altogether. Another way to reduce the amount of sugar when cooking and baking is to add lemon or orange zest, but make sure to use organic fruit, as pesticides and chemicals can be concentrated in the skin. As your taste buds grow accustomed to doing without the very powerful taste of refined sugar, you will come to appreciate the natural sweetness of vegetables and fruits.

There is so much confusion around 'natural' sweeteners that I am going to cover the choices in more detail.

Fructose

You can buy fructose as a white powder, just like sucrose (table sugar), to add to food as a sweetener. As we've already discussed, many people think fructose is fine as it is the fruit sugar naturally found in fruit. The problem is that, when it is sold as a white powder, it is totally refined and all the goodness and fibre that would be in the fruit is absent.

Interestingly, fructose does not cause the release of insulin as sucrose and glucose do, so initially it was thought to be a healthy form of sugar. However, it has other negative effects on your health.

Fructose goes straight to your liver which has to metabolise it, in the same way as alcohol does.So it can make you gain weight, increase your appetite and also give you fat around the middle. Fructose interferes with your production of hormones like leptin, which should send you a signal telling you that you have eaten enough, and fructose can raise levels of a hunger hormone called ghrelin, increasing your appetite. Fructose is converted into unhealthy fats such as LDL ('bad') cholesterol and triglycerides. As we have seen in previous chapters, high levels of triglycerides (blood fats) are associated with heart disease, diabetes and fatty liver disease.

Starches supply glucose to your brain and muscles and, when they are unrefined, the glucose is released slowly. But fructose does not supply any energy at all to either your brain or your muscles; it is only stored as fat.

When fructose is consumed as part of fresh fruit, combined with the fibre and nutrients, it does not have the same effects on the liver as the powdered refined fructose, as it is released more slowly and generally eaten in small quantities.

Again, you need to read labels, because fructose can be used as a sweetener in many foods, instead of, or as well as, other forms of sugar. It can also be found in food supplements, especially if they are powders, in order to make the powder sweeter.

My view:
I would never use fructose as a sweetener. If it is naturally contained within the fruit then that is fine but I would not buy it as a white powder to add to food.

Agave

This sweetener has become very popular over the last few years. In theory, it should be a good natural sweetener as it comes from the agave plant in Mexico, where traditionally the sap would have been boiled for hours to obtain the sweet syrup. The problem is that when something is commercially produced corners are cut to make a product financially viable. To produce agave on a commercial scale, the agave is made from the starch of the root bulb and the final product is just refined fructose because it is made by the same process that converts corn starch into high fructose corn syrup. It is even said that the fructose content is higher than the high fructose corn syrup which has had such a bad press in America.

Some agave syrups look darker than the others and one could think that maybe the amber coloured one was a more natural or superior product. But it has been suggested that the colour is produced when the fructose is burned so maybe the darker syrup is not such a good choice.

There may be some companies who produce the agave syrup in the traditional way but it is not easy to tell given the marketing hype around the products. They would be definitely be more expensive because of time making the product and availability.

My view:
I would not recommend using agave as it could be up to 90% fructose and there doesn't seem to be a way of distinguishing whether the agave has been made in the traditional way or whether it is commercially produced.

Honey

Although this is a natural sweetener, you should only use it sparingly. Honey is a simple sugar, primarily made up of glucose and fructose, and so is absorbed into your blood stream quickly, hence it's not ideal if you're trying to control your blood sugar or lose weight. The fructose content can be up to 40 per cent in some honeys.

If you do use honey then avoid types which are 'blended' or the 'produce of more than one country' because they are often heated to temperatures as high as 71°C (160°F), which destroys their natural goodness.

Bees gather nectar from flowers to take back to the hive. Honey is often harvested from the hives in the autumn, which means that the bees will struggle without food over the winter. So the bees are fed a substitute for nectar which is white sugar dissolved in hot water. Some 'natural' beekeepers leave enough honey in the hive so the bees can feed until the spring. However commercial beekeepers look just at the financial cost because they can sell the honey for more than the sugar water costs to feed the bees over the winter.

So, in effect, you may not be buying 'pure' honey, even though it might say so on the label, because the sugar water gets mixed up with the honey in the hive and, basically, the raw material for the honey is simply white sugar.

In America, they have been using high fructose corn syrup (HFCS) instead of sugar water to feed bees over the winter because it is cheaper. There are concerns that HFCS may have a detrimental effect on the health of the bees. Hydroxymethylfurfural (HMF) is a heat-formed contaminant found in HFCS which is toxic to bees and can cause ulceration of their digestive tract[58]. It is suspected as one of the possible causes of the widespread death of bees.

Even just using sugar syrup can be a problem for the bees. If the syrup has been badly produced, it can still produce high levels of HMF. In Belgium, abnormal losses of honey bee colonies were seen in colonies fed with inverted beet sugar syrup which contained high concentrations of HMF. The authors of the research state: 'These losses suggest that HMF could be implicated in bee mortality, a topic that so far has received only little attention'[59].

It is impossible to tell from the honey label whether the bees have been fed sugar over the winter months. The UK Soil Association has standards for organic honey that determine what the bees can be fed and where the apiaries must be sited. However, as the Soil Association itself points out, 'these rules effectively mean that UK producers cannot produce organic honey'.

The rules regarding the siting of apiaries state that they must:

- Be on areas of land that are certified as organic.

- Ensure enough natural nectar, honeydew and pollen sources for bees and access to water.

- Be such that, within a radius of four miles from the apiary site, nectar and pollen sources consist essentially of organic crops and/or uncultivated areas (spontaneous vegetation) and crops not subject to the provisions of these standards but treated with low environmental impact methods such as those described in programmes developed under Regulation (EEC) No 2078/92 which cannot significantly affect the organic description of the beekeeping.

- Maintain enough distance, if necessary, from non-agricultural production sources that may lead to contamination, for example: urban centres, motorways, industrial areas, waste dumps or waste incinerators.

The National Organic Standards Board in America also has a number of criteria for certifying organic honey, including the siting of the apiaries. They also say that organic honey producers must ensure 'maintenance of adequate supplies of honey and pollen in the hive, including leaving hives with reserves of honey and pollen sufficient for the colony to survive the dormancy period' - so, basically, they can't be fed sugar syrup or HFCS[60].

In Chapter 5, I mentioned some research that showed that a substance called methylglyoxal (MG) made HDL ('good') cholesterol less effective. MG is formed from glucose in your body. So MG would seem not to be a good thing.

And yet in order for honey to be called Manuka honey it has to contain a certain amount of MG. It is thought that it is the high levels of MG naturally contained in Manuka honey that give it its antibacterial properties.

There is a ratings scale called UMF (Unique Manuka Factor) and Manuka honey is considered to have therapeutic benefits if it has a UMF over ten.

The biggest concern is that three times more jars of honey labelled as Manuka are being sold world-wide than being produced in New Zealand where the Manuka (tea tree) bush grows.

Honey has been used traditionally for many years to heal wounds and research has shown that Manuka honey is particularly beneficial for this[61].

Honey when used on wounds needs to be sterilised first because bacterial spores such as spores of Clostridium could occur in honey and then be transferred to open wounds. So you would use medicinal honey, not the honey you would have at home, to treat wounds.

MG is a precursor of the advanced glycation end-products (AGEs), mentioned before, which damage tissue, making you age faster on the inside and visibly look older on the outside. It is thought that both MG and AGEs play a role in the problems that diabetics have with poor wound healing. So there are concerns that using Manuka honey containing MG could delay wound healing in diabetics[62].

Other research says not, because Manuka honey contains other substances that counteract the effect of the MG and that diabetic ulcers have been healed using Manuka honey[63].

So, very confusing and I would always err on the side of caution and maybe use medicinal honey for wounds in general but not for someone with diabetes.

My view:
Not an ideal sweetener as it is a simple sugar and so will affect your blood glucose (sugar) quickly. If you are going to use honey, try to get organic if possible and use very sparingly.

Molasses

Molasses is the by-product of the process used to extract sugar from sugar cane or beet.

The sugar cane juice is boiled and sugar crystallised from it. The syrup that is left over is molasses. Normally, the sugar cane is boiled three times to remove as much sugar as possible and the molasses left over at the end of this third stage is called black strap molasses and is dark in colour, very syrupy and has the lowest amount of sugar but the highest quantities of vitamins and minerals. It is a good source of vitamin B6 and potassium and a very good source of magnesium and manganese.

About half of the sugar content is made up of fructose and glucose in equal amounts and the other half sucrose.

My view:
This has not been a sweetener that I have used, as it is a by-product of sugar extraction and, as a result, may have higher levels of the pesticides and other chemicals used in sugar cultivation and processing. It also has a very strong taste.

Xylitol

This is another sweetener that has gained in popularity over the last few years. It is sold as a white powder and is considered natural because it occurs naturally in plants. It is low in calories and does not need insulin to be metabolised in the body so it is very useful for diabetics. It also has benefits for dental health as it reduces caries. Its main side effects are diarrhoea and bloating as it is a sugar alcohol (polyol), and so ferments in the digestive system, and would not be recommended for anyone following the FODMAP diet for IBS.

Xylitol is found in the fibres of many plants, including sugar cane, corn cobs and birch. However, it requires a lot of refining to take it from the raw product to a white powder.

Basically, xylitol is made from the hydrogenation of a sugar called xylose, which is produced from the fibre of the plant. The word 'hydrogenation' rings warning bells as we have been moving away from hydrogenated fats over the years, after we found out about the health risks associated with them. There may be concerns about hydrogenated sugar in years to come.

The whole process of making xylitol is very complex and seems very far away from being 'natural' when nickel catalysts are needed in the process. Read this extract from a description of xylitol production.

'Xylitol can be prepared from xylose in a batchwise, three-phase hydrogenation process. High hydrogen pressures and relatively high temperatures are used. High pressure is needed in order to improve the solubility of hydrogen in bulk liquid, whereas the need for high temperatures derives from the fact that the reaction is very temperature-dependent: the hydrogenation velocity is considerably enhanced by increased temperature. A Rushton turbine impeller, coupled to a propeller mixer, was used to provide efficient gas dispersion and mixing of the reactor contents. Vigorous shaking is needed for elimination of the outer liquid-solid mass transfer. The catalyst used in the process was a Sponge Ni catalyst (commonly referred to as a Raney Nickel catalyst), and the most common solvent used was deionized water.

Earlier studies had shown that mixtures of solvents; such as 2-propanol-water, 2-pentanol-water and ethanol-octane-water; improve the velocity of hydrogenation. Nevertheless, their use can cause some practical difficulties due to the lower solubility of the xylose in these reaction media. Also, the mass transfer of the hydrogen from the gas to the liquid phase is faster when using the aqueous alcohol mixtures, since the solubility of hydrogen is much higher in alcohols than in water'[64].

My view:
I would not use xylitol as it requires far too much processing to be considered a natural product.

Sorbitol

Like xylitol, sorbitol is a sugar alcohol (polyol) and is often used in foods designed for diabetics because it requires little or no insulin. It is usually made from corn syrup. Sorbitol is found naturally in stone fruits such as prunes, plums and dates. Like some other sugar substitutes, it is a very heavily-processed product, including hydrogenation.

The side effects of sorbitol are similar to those for xylitol, in that it can cause diarrhoea because it stimulates bowel motion. Both sorbitol and xylitol can worsen IBS (Irritable Bowel Syndrome) and are contraindicated for this condition.

Erythritol is also a sugar alcohol like sorbitol but in small amounts it is supposed to cause less digestive upsets because it is a smaller molecule than sorbitol and 90 per cent of it is absorbed in the small intestine and then passed out through the urine. But there are individual variations with some people still experiencing stomach upsets or diarrhoea even with smallish amounts of erythritol.

My view:
I would not recommend using sorbitol or erythritol because of the negative effects on the digestive system and the fact that it is a heavily-processed sweetener.

Maple syrup

Maple syrup is made from the sap of maple trees by making a hole in the tree and collecting the syrup.

Research presented at the American Chemical Society's National Meeting in California in 2011 has suggested that maple syrup contains 34 beneficial compounds which have antioxidant and anti-inflammatory properties. A number of the syrup's antioxidant polyphenols inhibit the enzyme that converts carbohydrates to sugar, which is relevant to type 2 diabetes and weight gain. The research also showed that many of the antioxidants found in maple syrup, which can help prevent the ageing of our body's cells, aren't found in other natural sweeteners[65].

Maple syrup is the natural sweetener usually recommended for IBS sufferers as it causes the least problems with digestion and is included in the FODMAP diet, which restricts those foods that are highly fermentable in the intestines, in order to reduce the amount of bloating, flatulence, cramping and diarrhoea. So it would be one of the best sweeteners if you get these symptoms.

Maple syrup contains significant amounts of zinc and manganese and 15 times more calcium than honey. It is made up of primarily sucrose and very small amounts of fructose and glucose[66].

Beware maple syrup labelled as 'maple-flavoured syrup' rather than just 'maple syrup', as this won't be pure maple syrup. In fact, it may not contain any maple syrup at all. Ingredients of one of these maple flavoured syrups includes invert sugar syrup, colour (150d) and maple flavouring, while another one has water (the first ingredient), caramel colour, alcohol, vanilla extract (vanilla bean extractives in water), alcohol and corn syrup, molasses solids, corn syrup solids, natural and artificial flavour, sugar and sulphiting agents. That is why it is so important to read labels: you have to know what you are putting into your body. We will discuss this in more detail later.

Real maple syrup will be more expensive but bear in mind you will only be using small amounts.

My view:
I do use real maple syrup as a natural sweetener and I always buy organic where possible. I use it in cakes and to drizzle over the top of crumbles to give it a lovely browned effect.

Chloe Archer
Perms Consultant

T: 0207 828 2691
E: chloe.archer@reedglobal.com

The Peak
5 Wilton Road
Victoria
London
SW1V 1AN

reedglobal.com/accountancy

REED
ACCOUNTANCY

Accountancy, Actuarial, Administration,
Banking, Customer Services, Education,
Engineering, Expro, Finance, Health
& Care, Hospitality & Leisure, Human
Resources, Insurance, Management,
Marketing & Creative, Mortgages,
Property & Construction,
Procurement & Supply Chain, Retail,
Sales, Scientific, Technology.

Barley malt syrup

This is an unrefined natural sweetener produced from sprouted barley malt, which is dried and then cooked, sometimes called Barley Malt Extract. The liquid is then filtered and reduced down to the required consistency. It is thick and dark brown and makes wonderful flapjacks. It is a reasonably good source of some minerals and vitamins and contains almost no fructose or sucrose.

My view:
Barley malt syrup is a good choice as a natural sweetener. It has a malty taste so does not work well, taste-wise, in all recipes but, as I mentioned, brilliant for using in flapjacks where the malt is an added benefit.

Brown rice syrup

This syrup is a natural sweetener, available in most health food shops, also called rice malt syrup. Brown rice syrup contains three sugars – maltotriose, maltose and glucose. Cheaper versions are made from cooked brown rice cultured with enzymes to turn the starches in the rice into sugar. Others use sprouted grains that release the enzymes that breakdown the grain into maltose and other sugars. I would suggest buying an organic version, as it is more like to be made from sprouted grain. Also brown rice syrup doesn't contain any fructose, which is a good thing.

My view:
I personally would use organic brown rice syrup as a sweetener. It does tend to change the texture of baked foods, so is best used where a little crunch is of benefit. This makes it a good choice for a crumble, flapjack or healthy granola, in small amounts.

Stevia

Stevia is derived from the leaves of a South American plant of the same name. It has been used for centuries as a sweetener in South America and for 40 years in Japan. In 2011 it was approved for use in the EU. Stevia is 2-300 times sweeter than table sugar (sucrose).

Unfortunately, there are a couple of problems with stevia. Read labels very carefully as some products can contain dextrose and flavourings. You need a product that is 100 per cent stevia.

As stevia is not absorbed through the digestive tract, it is considered to have no calories, so it appears a good choice for weight loss. However, although pure stevia is more natural than artificial sweeteners, it still primes your body to expect a corresponding amount of calories for the sweetness. When that calorie hit doesn't happen, your body will send you off to get the calories from somewhere else, increasing your appetite and causing weight gain.

It has a slightly bitter aftertaste for most people, which is why it is often mixed with other sweeteners, especially in soft drinks and processed foods.

My view:
You could use stevia as a sweetener as long as you use it in moderation and it is just stevia in the product. Not everyone likes the taste and it is not a sweetener I have used at all.

Whole cane sugar

Adding to the confusion, there is another type of sugar you might find in products or sold separately to be added to food. The problem with refined sugar of any version is that it has no nutritional value because all the vitamins, minerals and other valuable nutrients have been lost in the processing.

Sugar cane itself, in its natural state (before any refining or processing), contains vitamins such as the B vitamins and vitamins A and C and also minerals such as calcium, chromium, zinc and magnesium. It also contains fibre, as any plant does, and polyphenol compounds that have antioxidant benefits (they are also found in green tea).

The juice is pressed from the sugar cane, heated over low heat and then dried and granulated. The molasses is separated from the sugar and it keeps all the nutrients intact because it has not been refined or subject to high heat. It is also sometimes known by its Portuguese name rapadura and also known as jaggery in Asia.

My view:
This would be the natural unrefined form of sugar and would really be the best way to eat or drink it. And, because it is in its whole form rather than refined, it would be absorbed more slowly into your bloodstream.

Evaporated cane juice

You may have noticed this newish ingredient in many 'natural' products and thought it a better alternative to sugar, as it sounds more 'natural'. However, the term is very misleading. The FDA in America has sent out warning letters to food companies saying not to use the term Evaporated Cane Juice (ECJ) because it is misleading and false as it is not a 'juice' at all but a sugar syrup.

The FDA is suggesting that food companies should call the ingredient 'dried cane syrup' or 'sugar cane syrup'.

ECJ is partially purified sugar so it is not quite as refined as sugar but the bottom line is that it's still sugar and will have very similar effects on your body as ordinary sugar. Supporters of ECJ say that because it is not as refined as ordinary sugar there are some nutrients left but they occur in such small quantities that they are irrelevant.

In countries around the world where they grow sugar cane they often will sell unrefined sugar cane juice. This is completely different from ECJ and it is where the juice is extracted, either manually or electrically, through crushing sugar cane and serving the drink with lemon or ginger.

My view:
Avoid products that contain evaporated cane juice as you are really just eating processed sugar.

Palm sugar

Palm sugar can also be known as jaggery but, instead of being made from sugar cane, it is made from the palm tree and, in particular, the palmyra palm tree. The palm flowers are tapped to release the juice, which is then boiled down to produce the syrup, which is then be allowed to crystallise.

It is a traditional Ayurvedic ingredient and contains good amounts of B vitamins (including a plant source of B12). It has a low glycaemic index (40) and it is suggested that is suitable for diabetics.

It is similar to coconut sugar (see below) but is made from the palm tree rather than the coconut tree.

My view:
A good natural sweetener and a nice alternative to sugar, can be used in cooking as well as drinks.

Coconut sugar

This sweetener is also known as coconut palm sugar and is produced from the sap of the flower buds of the coconut tree. It is found in liquid form as a syrup, as well as crystals. Coconut syrup is also known as coconut nectar and coconut blossom syrup.

To obtain the sap, the tree is tapped, as in the palm sugar, and minimally heated in order to allow moisture to evaporate to form the syrup. When the syrup cools down it crystalises.

Like palm sugar, coconut sugar is rich in nutrients such as the B vitamins, magnesium, calcium, potassium, zinc, 17 amino acids, short chain fatty acids, polyphenols and antioxidants; plus it has a nearly neutral pH. It also contains inulin which, like FOS, is a prebiotic and helps to feed beneficial bacteria.

Most information says coconut sugar has a low glycemic index of 35 but this was a study of just 10 volunteers. Research in 2014 from the University of Sydney shows a GI of 54[67], while white sugar has a GI of 65.

There are mixed opinions about the sustainability of coconut sugar. Some people are suggesting that because the sugar is made from the sap of the flower bud of the coconut tree, that once the sap has been collected, the tree can no long produce coconuts. So all the other valuable foods we get from the coconut tree - coconut oil, desiccated coconut, coconut milk and cream - would be lost[68].

Other people are saying that it is possible to produce both sap for making coconut sugar and coconuts from the same tree. That it just requires the coconut sap to be tapped in the first half of the coconut blossom and then letting the remaining half of the blossoms to mature into coconuts. It means that the coconut yields are about 50 per cent lower than when the trees are not tapped but it has been pointed out that this technique is feasible and very profitable for small producers. Using this kind of technique (producing both coconuts and sugar), small scale coconut farmers can have incomes nearly ten times higher per year than if they just produce coconuts and not the sugar as well.

They also suggest that tapping can stimulate fruit production so a young coconut tree tapped for 6-12 months for sugar production will produce more coconuts, sometimes up to three times more than if untapped[69].

As this last information is coming from the Food and Agriculture Organisation of the United Nations this would seem more plausible and would indicate that coconut sugar is a sustainable sweetener.

My view:
I have not used coconut sugar myself but it is supposed to taste like brown sugar and you would use it exactly the same as sugar. I would suggest buying organic coconut sugar.

Yacon syrup

This is a sweetener made from the sweet root of the yacon, which is a member of the sunflower family, also known as the Peruvian ground apple. It tastes like a cross between an apple and a pear. Yacon contains good amounts of a prebiotic called FOS (fructooligosaccharide), which helps to feed the beneficial bacteria in the digestive system. Prebiotics are not digested in the small intestines and make their way to the bowel to be used by the beneficial bacteria. Yacon also contains good amounts of vitamins and minerals. It is low GI, can help to lower glucose levels and is said to be fine for diabetics to use[70,71]. It is traditionally made without chemicals using evaporation, like maple syrup.

My view:
I would recommend this as a sweetener although I have not tried it yet. It can be used instead of a liquid sweetener such as honey and also in baking. Choose an organic variety. It may not be suitable for people with IBS due to its high FOS content.

Artificial sweeteners

Many people use artificial sweeteners as a substitute for sugar to help control their weight because, in strict opposition to sugar, artificial sweeteners have no calories. Ironically, artificial sweeteners can actually cause weight gain and will increase your appetite[72]. Bottom line? They make you eat more.

When you eat something sweet it usually comes with a bulk of calories. But artificial sweeteners have no calories so your body sends you off to find calories somewhere else. It does this by increasing your appetite and giving you cravings.

Sugar activates the sweet receptors on your tongue and increases dopamine in your brain, and the artificial sweeteners also have this effect. But sugar has a secondary effect when it causes an increase in glucose. Artificial sweeteners have no effect on your blood sugar or may even give you low blood sugar (hypoglycaemia) which leaves you feeling hungry and unsatisfied with what you have eaten, making you eat more the next time.

When rats are fed artificial sweeteners they take in more calories, weigh more and, even more worryingly, this weight is made up of an increase in body fat percentage. The researchers commented: 'These results suggest that consumption of products containing artificial sweeteners may lead to increased body weight and obesity by interfering with fundamental homeostatic, physiological processes.' Basically, the artificial sweeteners change the animals' inner control of knowing when they have had enough to eat[73].

Two groups of rats were given exactly the same amount of calories, but one group was given either saccharin or aspartame (artificial sweeteners) and the other group was given sugar (sucrose). The rats given the artificial sweeteners gained more weight than rats eating sugar[74]. So, even if you think you can control your appetite and you are not eating more when using artificial sweeteners, you are still going to gain weight.

We know that people who drink two or more diet drinks a day have waist circumference increases 500 per cent greater than people who don't drink diet drinks[75].

However, it is not only your waistline you have to worry about with artificial sweeteners. The increased risk of developing a serious illness is the major problem. Artificial sweeteners increase your risk of type 2 diabetes, metabolic syndrome (which causes a number of problems such as high cholesterol and high blood pressure) and heart disease. Scientists go further and say that these sweeteners have the effect of 'inducing metabolic derangements'[76]. They are altering how your body functions, which then puts you at risk of major life-threatening illnesses.

The suggestion is that artificial sweeteners (or non-caloric artificial sweeteners as they are often called) are causing glucose intolerance by altering the beneficial bacteria in the gut[77]. We already know that gut bacteria have a role to play in insulin resistance, obesity, non-alcohol fatty liver disease and type 2 diabetes[78] and that there is a difference in the gut bacteria composition in normal and overweight people[79].

There are a number of different artificial sweeteners including aspartame, saccharin, acesulfame-K and sucralose. I would strongly suggest you avoid them all. Let's look at why.

Aspartame

Aspartame was discovered by two scientists in the 1960s. They were working on an anti-ulcer drug and found that aspartame had a sweet taste. It is up to 200 times sweeter than sugar (sucrose).

Aspartame is derived from two amino acids, aspartic acid and phenylalanine. When aspartame is digested, it releases methanol and two amino acids, aspartic acid and phenylalanine, into your body. Methanol converts to formaldehyde and then to formate or formic acid. Amino acids are fundamental constituents of all proteins and they interact with each other. Amino acids are normally ingested in small quantities in proteins and in combination with other amino acids. In this case, however, aspartic acid and phenylalanine are being ingested on their own and in much larger quantities. The result is that they can unbalance the metabolism of amino acids in the brain.

Removing aspartame and also MSG from the diet for only four weeks in patients who had IBS and fibromyalgia resulted in 84 per cent of patients saying that over 30 per cent of their symptoms had been resolved. It is thought that both MSG and aspartame can over-stimulate nerve cells, so eliminating them from the diet could help in conditions where pain or hypersensitivity to pain is a predominant symptom[80].

Recent news from the European Food Safety Authority (EFSA) has concluded that aspartame is safe and poses no threat to health. The EFSA says that aspartame is safe at the current levels of exposure which are set at 40mg per kg of body weight per day. However, it has also been suggested that the EFSA panel was dominated by experts linked to manufacturers and previous supporters of aspartame.

My view:
Avoid at all costs.

Saccharin

Saccharin is most often thought of as the first artificial sweetener. It is made from petroleum materials. It is about 300 times sweeter than sugar (sucrose).

There have been a number of health scares concerning saccharin over the years, for example an increased risk of bladder cancer. However, the research has been conducted on animals and it is thought that the results do not apply to humans.

My view:
Even though there is not a lot of consensus about the health scares, this is an artificial sweetener, so avoid completely.

Sucralose

Sucralose is made by chlorinating sucrose (sugar). It is 600 times sweeter than sugar. Only about 15 per cent of the sucralose is absorbed by your body and the rest is passed out unchanged. So there have been concerns because sucralose has been detected in municipal effluents and surface waters both in Europe and the US. The concern is whether sucralose in the environment could have a toxic effect on animals, particularly those in an aquatic environment.

Sucralose is highly soluble in water and degrades very slowly which is why it has been detected in water. At the moment, research tends to the view that it is not affecting the aquatic wildlife[81] in terms of survival, growth and reproduction of algae, crustaceans, fish and plants. However, some studies have reported physiological and locomotion behavioural changes in certain aquatic organisms. Daphnia, a freshwater flea, when exposed to sucralose, swims at a different height and increased speed while gammarids, which are small crustaceans, take longer to reach food and shelter. The researchers suggest that 'regardless if these behavioural responses were initiated via traditional toxic mechanisms or stimulatory effects, they should be considered as a warning, since exposed organisms may diverge from normal behaviour, which ultimately can have ecological consequences'[82].

The other controversy concerning sucralose is that it has been marketed as being 'made from sugar, so it tastes like sugar'. Sugar is certainly used as the starting point, but the end product does not contain sugar. The Sugar Association in the US representing the sugar cane and sugar beet farmers filed claims against the manufacturers of sucralose as they thought that this was false-advertising and in France the slogan is banned. In America the slogan is now: 'It's made from sugar. It tastes like sugar. But it's not sugar.'

My view:
Avoid as it is chlorinated sugar and also avoid because of the environmental impact.

As you will have seen, there is a bewildering array of sweeteners on offer. My feeling? Choose and use wisely. Quite apart from any health issues individual products have, they could all encourage a sweet tooth, tempting your taste buds to want more sweetness in your food.

In the next chapter we'll look at how it isn't as simple as just choosing which (if any) sugars or sweeteners you buy to add to your food. Sugar and sweeteners are already in a vast proportion of the foods you buy.

CHAPTER 12

Reading Food Labels

Don't believe the hype.

This is the main message of this chapter. You can't trust food producers and shops. You need to become a label reader to understand what is in the food you eat. Truly, don't fall for the marketing hype on the front of the packet.

Breakfast cereals are one of the worst culprits of misdirection regarding the ingredients in the packet. Reading the information on the front of a packet of cereal you could easily believe that it's a really healthy choice. It could have the words 'fortified with vitamins' blazing across the packet, in order to bump up the nutritional benefits. It could say 'low fat' urging you to think that this constitutes a healthy breakfast but grains like corn are naturally low fat anyway. The cereal might say 'high in fibre' but refined bran may simply have been added to increase the fibre content rather than it being the natural fibre contained in the grain. They also might have cartoon or film characters on the packet for 'pester' appeal with children.

Reading the food label

There are certain things that *have* to appear on a food label. These include:

- The name under which the product is sold.

- A list of ingredients, in order of predominance. In other words, the first ingredient in the list will be the predominant ingredient.

- The quantity of certain ingredients and net quantity.

- A use by date.

- Any special storage instructions or conditions of use.

- The name or business name and address of the manufacturer or packager, or of a seller within the European Union.

- The place of origin of the foodstuff.

- Instructions for use where necessary.

- Beverages with over 1.2 per cent alcohol by volume must declare actual alcoholic strength.

When I look at a label, I look firstly at the nutrition information which is usually in a table format - see the example below. This can appear really confusing but you want just to focus on two things in the table, the serving size and the sugars.

The serving size on this label, which is a breakfast cereal, says 30g but it is likely you would put more in the bowl. The other important part to look at is the sugar content which says 11g for a 30g serving size. 4g of sugar is equal to one teaspoon so in that small serving size of 30g there are nearly three teaspoons of sugar. Of course, many people then sprinkle more sugar on the top of their breakfast cereal!

	Typical value per 100g	30g serving with 125ml of semi skimmed milk			
ENERGY	160 6kJ 379 kcal	733 kJ 173 kcal	VITAMINS:	(% RDA)	(% RDA)
PROTEIN	14g	9g	VITAMIN C	8.3 µg (167)	2.5 µg (50)
			VITAMIN D	134 mg (167)	42 mg (52)
CARBOHYDRATE	76g	29g	THIAMIN (B₁)	1.8 mg (167)	0.6 mg (55)
of which sugars	17g	11g	RIBOFLAVIN (B₂)	2.3 mg (167)	1mg (72)
starch	59g	18g	NIACIN	26.7 mg (167)	8.2 mg (51)
FAT	1.5g	2.5g	VITAMIN (B₆)	2.3 mg (167)	0.8 mg (56)
of which saturates	0.5g	1.5g	FOLIC ACID	334 µg (167)	108 µg (54)
FIBRE	2.5g	2.5g	VITAMIN B₁₂	4.2 µg (167)	1.8 µg (71)
SODIUM	0.45g	0.2g	MINERALS		
SALT	1.15g	0.5g	IRON	11.6 mg (83)	3.5 mg (25)

This information can cause confusion. In 100g of cornflakes there can be 18g of sugar (just over four teaspoons) according to the label, whereas a muesli which contains no added sugar has 12.2g of sugar per 100g serving. That is because the muesli can contain raisins or other dried fruits which naturally contain sugar.

The label above does not distinguish between added sugar and sugar that is naturally contained within the food. Legislation does not insist on this and the food industry doesn't want this to change.

However, in America there are plans to pass a bill to change food labels to show how much refined sugar is added to the product rather than just showing the total sugar content.

The most important part of the food label that I check is the ingredient list. This tells me exactly what is in the food. Anything ending in 'ose' (glucose, sucrose, fructose, lactose, maltose) - is a form of sugar, as are honey, agave, molasses and syrups like corn and rice syrup, not forgetting glucose-fructose syrup (high fructose corn syrup). The nearer to the beginning of the ingredient list, the more of that ingredient is in the produce.

To give an example, let's look at one packet of popular jellies. These are the ingredients listed on the packet:

Glucose Syrup, Sugar, Dextrose, Gelatine, Citric Acid, Caramelised Sugar Syrup, Flavourings, Fruit & Plant Concentrates (Apple, Aronia, Blackcurrant, Elderberry, Grape, Kiwi, Lemon, Mango, Nettle, Orange, Passion Fruit, Spinach), Colours (Carmine, Copper Complexes of Chlorophyll), Glazing Agents (Vegetable Oil, Beeswax, Carnauba Wax), Invert Sugar Syrup, Fruit Extract (Carob).

One hundred grammes of these jellies gives 63.4g of sugar; that is nearly 16 teaspoons. As glucose syrup, sugar and dextrose are the first three ingredients, the jellies are mainly made up of these - there is not that much else in the product. The next ingredient listed is gelatine. Gelatine is extracted from the skin, boiled crushed horn, hoof and bones, connective tissues, organs and some intestines of cattle, chicken, pigs and horses. After that it is just flavourings and glazing agents. Your eye could easily be drawn to all those 'healthy' fruits but, in reality, there are barely any in the jellies.

Even something that might appear to be a healthy food, such as yogurt, can contain up to eight teaspoons of sugar. Look at the ingredients in this yogurt which contains 25.5g of sugar per pot - six teaspoons.

Yogurt, Sugar, Water, Cocoa Butter, Milk Powder, Flour (Rice, Wheat, Maize), Cocoa Mass, Modified Maize Starch, Whey Powder, Lactose, Flavourings, Wheat Starch, Caramel, Stabilisers: Pectins, Acacia Gum; Emulsifier: Soya Lecithins; Salt, Barley Malt, Vegetable Fat).

Become a label reader. I know it takes a bit of time at first but, once you learn which brands don't contain added refined sugars, then your shopping becomes routine.

By now you must be wondering what is left that you can eat freely! Rest assured that you can eat a wide, varied and delicious diet without compromising your health and wellbeing. In the next chapter I'll teach you how to balance your cravings and start a whole new regime that will support your health, your weight, your fitness and even your looks.

CHAPTER 13

What to Eat to Stop Sugar Cravings

In my clinic, people often say to me that they will never be able to give up sugar. However, you'd be surprised how quickly your taste buds change and how you come to appreciate the sweetness of other foods such as roasted sweet potatoes and carrots.

I would suggest that you have a good spring clean of your food cupboards and discard anything containing sugar. It's tempting to give away food if the sell by date is fine but do you really want to encourage anyone else to eat sugar? Bin it.

When I started out in the nutrition field over 30 years ago, it was much harder for people as there simply weren't the choices there are now. Nowadays if, say, you don't have time to make your own salad dressing, there will usually be an alternative in the shops that you can use, avoiding ones with high levels of sugar and sweeteners. The same goes for spaghetti sauces and mayonnaise. It is just a question of getting used to buying different brands. You may find that your local health food shop will stock some alternatives for foods that you regularly buy that are sugar-free (with no artificial sweeteners added) and that will taste quite delicious.

I have included some sugar-free recipes in this book. I have also included some savoury ones as you may be surprised to find just how much sugar is in the savoury foods you eat.

Mainly, I want to show you that you can have sweet foods that are not laden with an ingredient that is full of calories and has no nutritional value.

Eat little and often

To keep your blood sugar balanced and to avoid the dips (low blood sugar, hypoglycaemia) that will send you racing off to get a quick fix with a chocolate bar or a packet of biscuits, make sure that you are eating little and often.

My recommendation is have a good breakfast, lunch and dinner and also to include a mid-morning and a mid-afternoon snack. Don't go longer than three hours without eating (this is especially vital for women) or your blood sugar levels will drop too low and your body will give you a craving for something sweet to rectify the drop quickly.

If you miss breakfast you are setting yourself up to fail because by 11am you will be craving a coffee and a Danish because your blood sugar will have dropped so low. Remember that breakfast means 'breaking the fast'. You have not eaten since dinner the night before and that first meal of the day is the one that breaks the fast. Of course it needs to be a good breakfast and so I have given suggestions. If you opt for a sugary breakfast cereal, this will give a quick rise in blood sugar followed by a drop soon afterwards, giving you the feeling that you need something else, another quick fix to keep you going and so it goes on.

Intermittent fasting and the 5:2 diet

A recent trend has been to follow diets which require you to fast, such as the 5:2 alternate or intermittent fasting. I would suggest you avoid these while you are adjusting to not eating sugar.

Normally, I would recommend that women eat around 2,000 calories a day and men 2,500 but the important points are the quality of those calories (avoiding sugar and refined carbohydrates). You want to avoid having blood sugar highs and lows which not only control the release of insulin in your body but also that of the stress hormones adrenaline and cortisol.

Why don't I recommend variations on intermittent fasting? First of all, it is not suitable for everyone. If you are pregnant, breast feeding, diabetic, under 18 or have a history of an eating disorder then you shouldn't follow this regime. Equally fasting isn't for you if you are prone to blood sugar swings where you feel weak, headachey, dizzy or light headed when you don't eat. I also don't think it is beneficial for anyone suffering from chronic fatigue or if you are very stressed. Your body perceives fasting as a form of stress, because it detects that there is a shortage of food, which is a survival issue, life or death. So if you are already stressed or fatigued you shouldn't add another stress, lack of food, to your body. Also if you do a lot of exercise or are training for an event then you would need to think carefully about doing this kind of diet.

Apart from all this, there are many variations to this diet and nobody yet is clear which regime works the best. 5:2 fasting is where you fast on two days a week and again it is not clear whether it is better if the two days are consecutive or broken up and also whether it needs to be complete fasting (just taking water) or cutting down to 600 calories for men and 500 calories for women on the fasting days. If you follow the 5:2 fast with restricted calories, there is no definite research yet to say whether it is better to have all the calories in one meal or spread out throughout the day.

Other regimes suggest alternate day fasting, where you are fasting every other day of the week.

On non-fasting days, no matter what regime you are following the suggestion is that you can eat anything and how much you want.

I think this kind of diet is harder for women than men because we are much more susceptible to blood sugar fluctuations and this can be even harder depending on which part of the menstrual cycle you are in.

I am also concerned that, often, these types of diets suggest you rely on black coffee, tea or diet drinks to get you through the fasting days. If you use caffeine in this way then you are going to be living on adrenaline for the fasting days and that is not healthy. Many people have also found that on the non-fasting days they end up over-indulging in unhealthy foods and more calories to compensate for the fasting days. My major concern is that this type of fasting diet could tip some people into having an eating disorder.

Having caffeine can also make you crave sugar so it would be better to limit caffeine in order to make it easier to stop the sugar.

Weaning yourself off sugar

I would suggest you follow these simple steps to make coming off sugar easier. You could take these steps one week at a time or a day at a time. It really depends on your personality. It is a bit like someone giving up smoking, some people would rather just stop; others gradually reduce. The choice is yours.

1. First of all, take out of your diet all the savoury foods that contain added sugar. This might be as simple as just changing the brand so you keep the same food but the ingredients are healthier. Or you might have to ditch that food, if there isn't an alternate, or make it yourself. Foods to think about are tomato (spaghetti) sauces, mayonnaise, salad dressings, baked beans and soups. So, for example, a shop-bought sweet chilli sauce has sugar as the first ingredient. I would suggest that, if you still want to use this kind of sauce, to make it yourself and add a little pure maple syrup to give that sweet taste.

2. The next step is to stop adding sugar to your hot drinks and other foods. Some people will sprinkle sugar on to their cereal in the morning when there is already a lot of sugar added to it (remember, read those packets). This is similar to people who sprinkle salt on their food before tasting it, when it might be salty enough. Wean yourself off added sugar, gradually diminishing the amount you use each day over a period of days or maybe weeks.

3. Next, have a look at the sweet foods you are eating on a regular basis that contain added or hidden sugar. You might think fruit yogurt that says 'live' on the tub is healthy but bear in mind, as we have seen, that it can contain up to eight teaspoons of sugar. Buy natural organic yogurt and drop in or blend in your own fruit, fresh or frozen. Alternatively, choose children's yogurts sweetened with fruit juice (but do check the label).

   Those cereal bars that seem 'natural' may be loaded with sugar. Sugar is, technically, natural so the marketing is correct but, nonetheless, it is not good for you. There are usually alternate brands you can buy that will be sugar-free, using naturally sweet ingredients such as dates and dried fruits.

   There may be some foods that have no alternative. My suggestion for these is to think of the 80/20 rule. This states that, if you are eating well 80 per cent of the time, it's okay to indulge for the remaining 20 per cent. So the occasional slice of chocolate cake at a party is not a big deal; it is what you are eating and drinking on a daily basis that counts.

4. Think about the amount of caffeine you are drinking in coffee, tea, colas and energy drinks. They will cause a similar roller coaster effect to sugar and cause the release of the stress hormones, adrenaline and cortisol. They are classed as stimulants. Because they can cause a drop in blood sugar, they can also trigger either sugar cravings or an increase in appetite in general. Also, when you are changing habits there may be some that are natural stable-mates, such as tea and biscuits, or coffee and a chocolate bar. So it can be easier to break a habit by breaking the association. If you are not having the cup of coffee, you might not think about having the chocolate bar.

5. I have not mentioned alcohol in this book but it does have an effect on your blood sugar. Think about the types of alcohol and which have a lower sugar content. You might want to make some changes. Red wine is thought to be one of the healthiest alcoholic drinks because of its high content of antioxidants but you could also have white wine and make it into a spritzer by adding mineral water, so you end up drinking less alcohol. Also the drier the wine, the less sugar, so a dry white is a better option. Fortified wines, such as sherry and port, are high in sugar.

   Spirits are considered 'better' because they do not contain sugar. With spirits the bigger concern is what they are mixed with, as the mixers can contain sugar. Beer contains a lot of carbohydrate. Needless to say, liqueur spirits such as Cointreau, Cherry Brandy and Drambuie contain a lot of sugar.

Add protein to carbohydrates

Carbohydrates will be broken down into sugar but, as mentioned before, the more unrefined the carbohydrate the slower this happens and the less effect on your blood sugar.

You can change an unrefined carbohydrate into an even slower releasing one by adding protein as you eat it.

So, if you're having porridge you could add ground nuts and seeds (vegetable protein) and if you are having a jacket potato then you could add tuna (animal protein). You could also sprinkle cinnamon on your porridge along with the ground nuts and seeds. Cinnamon is helpful in balancing blood sugar, as it improves the transport of glucose into your cells.

Protein slows down the rate at which your stomach empties the food into the next part of the digestive tract and so it slows down the emptying of the carbohydrate too.

If you tend to crave something sweet after a meal, I would suggest you add more protein to that meal. When the meal contains a lot of refined starchy carbohydrates, like white rice or white pasta, this will cause your blood sugar to rise quickly. Then, when it drops you will crave something sweet. By adding in more protein (say, a piece of fish or nuts and seeds) or substituting a vegetable protein like quinoa for the white rice, you will slow down the rate of digestion and the rise in blood sugar.

Some of your cravings for something sweet after a meal may just be a habit, like always having a biscuit with your cup of tea. Maybe you generally have a dessert after your evening meal or a few squares of chocolate 'to round off the meal' and this has become habitual. So your body is not actually pushing you to have the sugar because your blood sugar has dropped but your mind has become used to having something sweet after the meal.

When you feel a craving for something sweet, just take a few moments and give yourself a bit of time to ask how you are really feeling.

Are you stressed?

Although a mug of coffee and a muffin might seem the ideal answer, it will actually make you feel more stressed over time because, as your blood drops from the sugar effect, more stress hormones are released. Your body will perceive that you are more stressed than you actually are because of the abundance of the stress hormones, adrenaline and cortisol, that have been released.

The answer is to use something else other than food to calm you down. That might be a short walk outside in the fresh air or having a bath with soothing essential oils. It might be having a cup of chamomile tea and reading a favourite magazine or, perhaps, going for a run or to an exercise class. Or it could be as simple as putting on your favourite music and dancing.

Are you eating without thinking?

This is now called mindless or unconscious eating, where you are grazing continuously or picking at biscuits or chocolates while watching television or looking at your PC or phone. You're not thinking about what is going into your mouth. You need to switch this around so it becomes mindful eating.

Always sit at a table to eat (don't eat at your desk or slumped watching television). Have no distractions so you can focus on your food. Sit upright to reset your posture. Smell your food first so your brain can send the correct enzymes to deal with it. Eat slowly, tasting the food in your mouth before you swallow it. Put your knife and fork down between mouthfuls. Keep checking in to discover if you are still hungry or starting to feel full. If you learn to check in with your body you can then decide if you really want to eat something or whether you are simply eating it 'because it was there'.

Are you thirsty rather than hungry?

This is interesting. Often the signals can become a little crossed. When you feel hungry and are craving something sweet, you may actually be dehydrated. Test this by having a glass of water or a herbal tea and see how you feel after that.

Are you comfort eating?

You might want something sweet because you are stressed, as we have already discussed, and want to eat sugary foods, thinking this 'comfort food' will calm you down. But comfort eating can also include eating sweet foods because you are bored, lonely, angry or sad. Ask yourself which emotion you are trying to dampen down by eating sugary foods. As with stress, try to find an activity that actually deals with the emotion, rather than squashing it down. Talking to a friend could help or consider seeing a counsellor or therapist to get to the bottom of your feelings of anger or sadness.

Are you eating too fast?

You might fancy something sweet and actually just one square of chocolate would satisfy your craving. Often, however, we eat really fast, often not even chewing properly, and then end up eating the whole bar. It takes your brain 20 minutes to register that you are full and satisfied so when you eat quickly you can eat a lot before your body will tell you that you have had enough. If you ate that one square of chocolate slowly, thinking mindfully about what you are eating, taking your time and chewing well, you might find that the one square was enough and the craving had gone. Some schools of thought say that you should chew each mouthful 20 to 40 times. That takes practice but it's worth cultivating.

Many people will find this gradual reduction in sugar consumption works just fine. However, you might want to take a more radical step and start your new sugar-light way of life with a completely fresh start. In the next chapter we will look at how to take a total sugar detox.

CHAPTER 14
The Five Day Sugar Detox

If you find the idea of slowly weaning yourself off sugar difficult, you may prefer a more radical approach. Some people find it is actually easier to cut out all sugar; to go on a sugar detox.

If you want to make a radical change to your health and wellbeing, this is a great way to kickstart your body's healing. In this chapter I will give you all the tools you need for a total sugar detox. It involves eliminating all added sugar, artificial sweeteners, fruit and starches for five days.

Look on this as a chance to rethink the way you eat; an opportunity to recalibrate your metabolism and a way of reprogramming your taste buds to appreciate a variety of tastes in your food, rather than just sweetness. In fact, it's a very real gift for your body, mind and mood.

If you stick to it, you will notice very distinct results. You will undoubtedly lose weight if you need to, but this is not a weight-loss regime – it's about gaining control over your sugar addictions. Sleep almost invariably improves, as do stress levels as your blood sugar and hormone levels start to balance. Your skin will look clearer and brighter, your face may well lose any puffiness and your eyes will become clearer. These are just the external benefits! Inside, your body will be heaving a deep sigh of relief as it is able to reduce inflammation and allow hormones to return to better balance.

You will have plenty to eat but you may still find it challenging, if you're accustomed to lots of sugary treats, and even if you eat a lot of fruit and starchy vegetables. But just think – it's only five days and you will feel absolutely incredible.

You may wonder why I eliminate caffeine from this regime when it need not involve sugar. As we've seen already in this book, many people with a sugar problem also have imbalances of their stress hormones. By removing caffeine, you can help to reset your stress hormones. Also, as we've already discussed, because drinks containing caffeine can cause a rise and then a drop in blood sugar, they can also trigger either sugar cravings or an increase in appetite in general.

When detoxing is not advised

A general cleanse like this is safe for most people. However I would not advise you to do it if you:

- Are pregnant or breast-feeding.
- Have an eating disorder.
- Are diabetic
- Are feeling unwell or under par, or are getting over an illness.

If you have a serious medical condition and if you are on any medication, please consult with a health-care practitioner before embarking on this.

Preparation

Choose a time for this detox when you don't have a lot of commitments. You will feel a little tired for the first few days so don't plan anything too strenuous. It's also great if you can schedule time off so you can incorporate some gentle exercise and feel-good sessions into your week. It can be tricky eating out on this regime so try to pick a time when you can prepare your own food. If you do need to go to work or eat on the go, you can make up pack lunches and snacks to take with you. Alternatively, you can always ask a restaurant for plain grilled fish with green vegetables, or an omelette and green salad.

I firmly advise you do as much as possible of your shopping in one trip, so you're not tempted by sweet purchases on lots of shopping trips.

Clear out your cupboards and fridge, to avoid temptation.

If you regularly drink black tea and coffee, wean yourself off it over a week or so before starting the detox (otherwise you may experience bad headaches as a withdrawal symptom).

Side effects

It's not uncommon to experience side effects with this type of detox. Don't be alarmed, it's just your body throwing off toxins. Common side effects include:

- Tiredness, heavy legs.
- Interrupted sleep.
- Headaches.
- Unusual bowel movements – either constipation or loose bowels.

- Light-headedness.

- Upset stomach.

- Furry tongue.

- Spots, rashes or pimples.

- Bad body odour and bad breath.

- Cravings, particularly for sweet flavours.

Most people who undertake this detox find they hit 'the hump' – usually on day three or four. You may feel physically or emotionally low – or both. Don't panic and don't give up – this is totally natural – and it shows the detox is really working! Just be very gentle on yourself and keep going. Soon after the 'hump' you will start to feel amazing.

Exercise

You should schedule in some exercise on this programme (it helps the detox effect) but keep it gentle for the initial stage. Think about things like yoga, Pilates, walking out in nature, swimming, gentle toning classes, rebounding (bouncing on a small trampoline). Keep it low-intensity as you are on a very low carb diet – and so you may not have the boundless energy you might usually have.

Once you start incorporating more carbohydrate into your diet, you can increase the amount and intensity of your exercise.

Psychology

Be gentle on yourself as you undergo this programme. From a very early age we have been taught that sugar equals love, comfort, rewards. Think about it – how often as a child were you given sweets or cakes as a prize or reward? 'If you eat up all your greens, you can have pudding' was a refrain that rang through many houses.

By the time we have grown up, the pattern is often set. We tend to associate sweets, chocolate, cakes and biscuits with relaxation, we reward ourselves with a cookie or a chocolate bar and we comfort ourselves with biscuits and ice cream. Remember that sugar has the same effect on the reward centres of the brain as opiates – no wonder it's so addictive. The problem is that, no matter how often you might say to yourself, 'this is crazy! Stop treating yourself with sugar', your brain simply won't take it in. This detox gives you the chance to break that pattern and to start to rewire your neural pathways so you can begin to reward yourself with choices that are cleaner, healthier, kinder to your body and mind.

This is why I strongly suggest you factor in some feel-good pampering sessions during the detox. If you pick carefully, not only do they give you a psychological 'reward', they can also support your detox. I recommend the following in particular:

- Bathing. Even if you're usually a power shower sort of person, make time for healing, soothing baths. Skin brush before your bath, using a natural bristle brush on dry skin, working from your extremities (fingers, toes) towards your heart. Add good quality aromatherapy blends, or mineral salts like Epsom salts. If you have the option of a spa day with a therapeutic bath and detox scrub, so much the better.

- Massage. All massage supports detoxing but some forms of massage are particularly effective. Look out for MLD (manual lymphatic drainage), deep tissue massage, clinical aromatherapy, myofascial and neuromuscular techniques.

- Steam baths and saunas. The skin is our largest organ of elimination and sweating out toxins is a great support for this programme. Do take it easy, though, if you're not used to heat.

The five day sugar detox

Your food list is more limited than normal but that doesn't mean your food needs to be boring.

FOODS YOU CAN EAT

- Green vegetables. Green really is your favourite colour on this detox. Load your diet with all types of green veg: bok choy, cabbage, kale, broccoli, courgettes, marrow, lettuce, rocket, green peppers, mangetout, beans, seaweeds, peas, broad beans, sugar snap peas.

- White vegetables. Cauliflower, garlic, onions, leeks, celery, asparagus, fennel.

- Purple vegetables. Aubergine, purple sprouted broccoli, red cabbage.

- Good quality protein. Fish, organic eggs, seafood, quinoa, nuts, seeds, beans, tofu.

- Avocado.

- Seeds and nuts (all types). Including nut butters (home-made or without added sugar) and nut milks (again, without any added sugar or sweeteners).

- Quinoa. Although this cooks up like rice it is actually a seed and not a grain. It is also a complete protein.

- Buckwheat. This is also a seed and the flour can be used too.

- Sprouted seeds and pulses.

- Miso.

- Coconut (fresh, oil, cream). You can use coconut oil for frying (as a fat that is solid at room temperature it does not degrade when heated to high temperatures).

- Herbal teas (nettle, peppermint, etc.). Not fruit teas.

- Herbs and spices.

- Olives and capers.

- Cider vinegar, olive oil, flaxseed oil (for dressings).

That really is it. You may be wondering why no starchy vegetables are included, such as carrots, parsnips, sweet potatoes and potatoes? These are excluded from this five day sugar detox because they are higher in carbohydrates (natural sugars) than the non-starchy vegetables mentioned in the list. Dairy is also excluded for the five days because most of the dairy products will contain lactose (milk sugar) and it is better to eliminate the different kinds of sugars.

Just for clarity, potatoes and sweet potatoes are not the same kind of plant. Potatoes belong to the Solanaceae family; which includes tomatoes, peppers and aubergines; and are in the same class of plants as deadly nightshade. Sweet potatoes are part of the Convolvulaceae family of plants and although similar to look at they are not yams which are part of the Dioscorea family.

Fruit is also excluded in the five day detox but if you want to add in some fruit then go for berries, as they will have the least amount of sugar. You can also use some tomatoes and mushrooms to add variety to the savoury food.

Let's look at some menu ideas.

BREAKFAST

Make this a good solid meal, so you start off the day with energy. Don't be tempted to skip breakfast.

- Chia seeds soaked in coconut milk with coconut cream and a sprinkle of dry roasted nuts and seeds.

- Poached egg and avocado.

- Scrambled eggs with salmon.

- Smoked haddock.

- Omelette with mixed vegetables and grilled tomatoes.

- Smoothie – consisting of 1 cup of frozen (or fresh) mixed berries, 5 fl oz of soya, almond or coconut milk or water, 5-6 fl oz water, 1 heaped tablespoon almonds and seeds (e.g. sesame, pumpkin, flaxseeds), 1 tablespoon flaxseed oil.

- Berry booster – blend together a 9oz pot of soya yogurt with 2 tablespoons mixed berries, 1 tablespoon of ground seeds/nuts and 1 tablespoon flaxseed oil.

- You can make other blends using the vegetables from the list on page 84 and make sure you add in some protein.

LUNCH

This should also be a sizeable meal, if possible. Your digestion is at its strongest at midday. I know that most people have to have the biggest meal of the day in the evening but see if you can change this just for the five days of the detox (but don't worry if you can't).

- Grilled sardines, herrings or mackerel fillets with green vegetables or salad.

- Broad bean, onion, broccoli and smoked tofu frittata.

- Tuna niçoise salad.

- Tuna (drain off the oil or use tuna in spring water), 2 pilchards, 4 sardines, 8oz prawns, lentils or mixed bean salad served with a large mixed salad of your choice. Use ½ tbsp flax oil as a dressing.

- 2 organic egg omelette (mushrooms, leek, herbs, garlic, tomato and grated courgette) with a large mixed salad. Use ½ tbsp flax oil as a dressing.

- Falafels and mixed salad on toasted pumpernickel bread.

SUPPER

Keep this meal light, warming and cooked. The less strain you put on your digestion at night, the better.

- Miso soup with vegetables and sesame tofu.

- Grilled plaice (or any fish of your choice, or tofu) with garlicky greens.

- Salmon with asparagus and leeks.

- Stir-fried prawns or tofu with a selection of stir-fried vegetables. Use ½ tbsp olive oil to stir-fry the food. Add tamari soya sauce plus mixed herbs to taste.

- Baked salmon or mackerel. Place 4oz of salmon or mackerel fillets into a casserole dish with lid. Brush with olive oil, season with black pepper and place a slice of lemon on top. Bake for 20-30 minutes at 375°F/190°C/gas mark 5. Serve with a mixed salad.

- Home-made soup with vegetables, beans or fish.

SNACKS

In order to keep your blood sugar levels balanced, you should also have two snacks a day – one mid-morning and one mid-afternoon. It needn't be large but should include enough protein to keep energy levels up and to prevent blood sugar dips. The following give a few ideas:

- Slices of fresh coconut.

- A small portion – around 25g – of dry-roasted seeds or nuts.

- A celery and nut butter 'sandwich' – a piece of celery sliced and filled with the pure nut butter of your choice (cashew, almond, peanut).

- Hummus with cucumber sticks.

- Kale 'chips' with sesame seeds.

TIPS

- Drink plenty of water in between meals. Keep a bottle with you at all times.

- Don't dilute your digestive juices by drinking water or any liquids with meals. If you want a drink then have a drink 30 minutes before or after food.

- Spice up meals with lots of herbs and spices. Apart from making meals more interesting, many herbs and spices have wonderful healing effects.

- Cook and eat mindfully. Take time to smell your food, taste it and chew it thoroughly. Put your knife and fork down between mouthfuls. Become aware of how your body feels.

HELP WITH DETOXING

While you are doing the five day detox you might like some help to make the process more effective. There are certain nutrients that can help your body detox more efficiently, while you are following the five day detox. Everyday life now bombards you with toxins and pollutants so your body can benefit from a helping hand to get rid of these toxins and give yourself a 'spring clean', no matter what the time of year.

Flaxseeds and psyllium are helpful in that they can support healthy bowel function, keeping you regular and eliminating waste and toxins. Psyllium, in particular, is known to help cleanse the colon and helps to 'unstick' old faecal matter. Chlorella can aid the elimination process and dandelion root is useful to support your liver function, as your liver is the waste disposal unit for your body.

Your digestive system contains billions of beneficial bacteria and they not only improve your nutrition because they help to manufacture the B vitamins and also vitamin K, but they also help to improve detoxification, by aiding digestion and stopping food sitting in your gut too long; putrefying, fermenting and producing toxins.

There are some good detox powders available and the one I use in the clinic is NHP's D-Tox Support which contains all the botanicals mentioned above plus probiotics. This powder can be mixed with water and drunk as it is or added to a smoothie or blend in the mornings.(see www.naturalhealthpractice.com).

NEXT STAGE

Congratulations! If you have followed the plan for five days, you should be feeling pretty amazing. Look in the mirror – can you see how much clearer your skin and eyes are? Your tongue is probably nice and pink and clean too. Your stomach should feel flatter, less bloated and doubtless, when you step on the scales, you will find you have lost quite a few pounds.

Now it's time to start to re-introduce natural sugars into your diet over the next few weeks. Please note, we're re-introducing natural sugars – foods that have a naturally higher sugar content – rather than adding sugars to your diet.

Your taste buds will have changed over the last five days so be prepared for a surprise. Even simple foods like an apple will seem really sweet. Take time to focus on each food as you re-introduce it – savour it, enjoy it.

I'd recommend introducing new foods one at a time. Pay attention to how your body feels with each one. If you feel uncomfortable with any foods (bloating, headaches, wind, aches, etc.), you may find you have an intolerance to that food and you are welcome to get in touch for help with this (see *Resources* page 143).

FIRST WEEK

Keep going with all the allowed foods you have been eating on the five day detox. In addition, you can add in starchy vegetables – parsnip, beetroot, carrot, sweet potato and squash (I would not include ordinary potatoes as the starch is digested quickly and so can affect blood sugar). Don't overdo it though – think in portion terms of no more than a cup per serving.

You can also add apples. Always make sure you have a little protein alongside (a few nuts or seeds maybe) to slow the sugar absorption.

Try and keep to your no-caffeine regime, if possible. If you absolutely need to add in ordinary tea and coffee then keep it black and no more than a cup a day. Ideally, however, keep going with your no-caffeine regime – your adrenal glands will thank you!

SECOND WEEK

Now you can add in a little dairy produce, if you want to. Pay close attention to how your body feels with this. Many people are intolerant of dairy and you may find it gives you headaches or increased mucous. Keep portions small, at least at first. I would suggest you try just adding in natural organic yogurt first of all as the beneficial bacteria (probiotics) will aid digestion of the lactose, the milk sugar, in the dairy food. Butter will not contain lactose (or only traces) as it is a fat and does not contain any carbohydrate. The dairy food with the highest content of lactose is milk. Cheese will contain much lower levels of lactose than milk because during the making of the cheese a certain amount of the lactose is converted to lactic acid. Some cheeses have very little lactose, especially those that are aged. If you look at the carbohydrate content on the label of the cheese under the heading 'of which sugars' this is will give you an idea of the lactose content.

You can also add in other fruits now, such as pears, but I would keep the tropical fruits likes mangos, papayas, bananas and grapes out at the moment.

THIRD WEEK

Now you can introduce wholegrains. Brown rice, wholegrain basmati rice, organic porridge oats, millet, barley, rye and spelt. Again, keep portions reasonable.

If you're really craving bread, then add in organic rye bread (the dark type).

FOURTH WEEK AND BEYOND

Now you can introduce other foods more freely. But, do take it easy. How are you feeling? I'm willing to bet you feel absolutely incredible. Don't undo all your good work. Your taste buds will have recalibrated so you won't crave very sweet tastes so much. A carrot or straight off the vine tomato should taste amazing! By all means include all kinds of fruit now – but always remember to take some protein alongside them, to stop those sugar spikes.

Yes, you can eat dried fruit – but you may find it too sickly now. And always include a protein so have nuts and raisins rather than raisins on their own.

Above all, listen to your body at every step along the way.

Should you take supplements while you're on this programme or, indeed, in general? Let's look at that question in the next chapter.

CHAPTER 15

Should You Take Supplements?

Do you really need to take supplements? We often hear that a 'well balanced diet' will contain everything we need and so supplements aren't necessary. I think the 'well balanced diet' is a myth and that nowadays food supplements can be an important addition to your diet. Certainly, while you are following the dietary recommendations in Chapter 13 and Chapter 14, to help you come off sugary foods and adjust your taste buds, there are certain nutrients that can be helpful.

Remember that sugar is 'empty calories' and has no nutritional value, so if you have been eating a sugar-heavy diet for some time you could have become depleted in certain key nutrients.

Another problem is that our food does not contain the nutrients it used to. Compared to the 1930s, the fruits and vegetables we eat contain an average of 20 per cent fewer minerals (magnesium 24 per cent, calcium 46 per cent, iron 27 per cent and zinc 59 per cent). Meat and dairy products are also depleted in nutrients, with iron being depleted by 47 per cent in meat and 60 per cent in milk, while the calcium loss in cheese goes up to 70 per cent for Parmesan cheese, according to the Independent Food Commission's *Food Magazine* (2005).

Food, especially fruits and vegetables, are now routinely flown hundreds or even thousands of miles and may have been sitting in warehouses for days before being delivered to the shops. This can cause the nutrients to be depleted.

Your three key supplements

First of all, I would suggest that you always take a good quality multivitamin and mineral as the foundation of your supplement programme. Choose a multi depending on your age, sex and what stage you are in your life. So you would choose a different multi if you are trying to get pregnant than if you want a multi for your general health and you would choose a different one if you are going through the menopause. Because you have different nutritional needs at different ages and stages of your life, you can use food supplements, along with a healthy diet, to help you meet those needs.

I use NHP (Natural Health Practice) supplements in my clinics along with other companies. I have formulated these supplements in association with

NHP so I know the quality is excellent. These are available to order online at www.naturalhealthpractice.com and see the *Resources* section of this book.

I would then suggest you take a vitamin C supplement alongside the multi, as there is never enough vitamin C in a multi, and thirdly I would suggest you use a separate omega 3 essential fatty acids supplement as well. These three products form the basis of a good supplement programme and are also beneficial for balancing blood sugar.

Vitamin C

Everyone tends to associate vitamin C with immune system function and also its antioxidant benefits. But it is an unusual nutrient, in that most animals can make vitamin C from glucose but we humans can't.

Vitamin C and glucose are very similar in their molecular structure and use the same transport systems in your body so they can end up competing with each other. If you have high levels of glucose (sugar) in your blood you can end up with low levels of vitamin C as the vitamin C will not be able to get into your cells. Both glucose and vitamin C need insulin to get into your cells

Insulin receptors pick up glucose and move it into your cells. Glucose has a stronger affinity for these insulin receptors than vitamin C, so glucose will always have priority over vitamin C as to which is transported. This means that the higher your blood glucose (sugar), the less vitamin C will make it into your cells.

The good news is that research has shown that giving a total of 1000mg of vitamin C a day to people with type 2 diabetes reduced both fasting blood sugar levels and HbA1c. The vitamin C also reduced LDL ('bad') cholesterol. It is interesting that 500mg of vitamin C a day was not enough to reduce fasting blood sugar, HbA1c or LDL[83].

I would suggest that you take 1000mg of vitamin C, split into two amounts of 500mg. The split is important as vitamin C is a water soluble nutrient so you lose it through your urine during the day. Make sure you are taking the alkaline form of vitamin C (as magnesium ascorbate) rather than the acidic form (ascorbic acid). The alkaline form is much gentler on your digestive system and it will be clear on the label as to what form the vitamin C is. NHP's Vitamin C Support is my recommendation.

Omega 3 fats

This may seem an unusual nutrient in terms of blood sugar balance but I can't stress enough how important it is to have good levels of omega 3. Omega 3 is an essential fatty acid which means that you cannot make it inside your body; the only way you can take it in is either through your food or via supplements. You get omega 3 fatty acids from oily fish, egg yolks, soya, flaxseeds and walnuts.

There are two issues surrounding omega 3 that you need to understand. The first is that we are not getting enough omega 3 in our diet but the second, and bigger, problem is that we are getting far too much omega 6.

Omega 6 fats are found in vegetable oils such as sunflower, corn and sesame seeds and also in evening primrose oil, which many women have taken for years. People often take a combined omega 3 and 6 supplement because they have read that we need a good balance of the omega fatty acids. This is true, but you have to take into account what your own levels are in the first place. It is no good adding in more omega 6 if you already have enough or maybe even too much in your body.

Signs of a lack of omega 3 fatty acids in your diet include dry skin, lifeless hair, cracked nails, fatigue, depression, dry eyes, lack of motivation, aching joints, difficulty in losing weight, forgetfulness and breast pain. If you have been following the myth that 'fat is fattening', then you could well be deficient in these essential omega 3s, especially if you have followed a low-fat or no fat diet.

We are now getting up to 25 times too much omega 6 from our diet than omega 3[84]. The problem with this imbalance is that having too much omega 6 causes inflammation in your body and, as I have already touched upon, it is now thought that inflammation is the cause of all our degenerative diseases including type 2 diabetes, heart disease, cancer and Alzheimer's.

On the other hand, when you eat omega 3 fats they are converted to substances that have an anti-inflammatory effect in your body. As well as their beneficial anti-inflammatory effects, omega 3 fats can help to balance your blood sugar, by reducing the amount of glucose in your blood, and even switch on anti-diabetic genes[85]. They can also improve levels of a substance called adiponectin, which is produced in your fat cells and can regulate glucose. Research is suggesting that this could then reduce the risk of type 2 diabetes and heart disease in people who are obese[86].

These omega 3 oils are so powerful in helping your cell receptors become sensitive to insulin that one study showed that substituting just seven per cent of dietary fat with omega 3 fatty acids for only four weeks, reversed the need for high levels of insulin to be released in response to a rise in blood sugar[87].

I would definitely suggest you find out whether you have an imbalance of omega 3 to 6 in your body. You can find out via a simple home finger prick blood test. See www.naturalhealthpractice.com.

Having the correct balance of omega 3 and omega 6 in your blood is important not only in terms of balancing blood sugar and controlling inflammation in obvious places like joints, bowels (e.g. inflammatory bowel disorders) and skin (problems like eczema) but also because research is now pointing out how important these omega 3s are to your brain function and to the prevention of dementia and Alzheimer's.

Excess omega 6 comes from obvious places, such as vegetable oils, which are found in a lot of prepared foods. However, a less obvious source of omega 6 essential fatty acids is from meat and chicken.

You may think you are making a healthier choice by buying corn-fed chicken because it sounds more 'natural'. However, truly free-roaming poultry would feed on a wide variety of foods such as plants, seeds, worms and bugs. Corn-fed chicken eat, obviously, just corn. They have lower levels of omega 3 and much higher levels of omega 6 in their meat, and also in their eggs, than chickens allowed to feed in the natural way. A healthy ratio of omega 3 to 6 in eggs would be 1:2 but with corn-fed chickens, eggs can have a ratio of 1:20. There is also the issue of corn-fed chickens being contaminated with pesticides from the corn.

The same issue occurs with grain fed cattle: Once again, you are consuming too much omega 6 and not enough omega 3[88]. In addition, the grain feeding of the cattle causes high levels of trans fats. These are the worst type of fats you can possibly eat as they can increase your risk of heart disease by boosting levels of bad cholesterol (LDL) while decreasing levels of good cholesterol (HDL). If you increase your consumption of trans fats by just two per cent you can increase your risk of heart disease by a massive 30 per cent. These fats can also block the absorption of the essential fats[89].

Trans fats harden cells so they can harden arteries but they can also harden your insulin receptors, making you more insulin resistant and increasing the risk of type 2 diabetes. Avoiding trans fats can reduce your risk of diabetes by 40 per cent.

Still not convinced? Trans fats can also make you put on weight around the middle of your body even if you are eating a low calorie diet[90].

Trans fats are found in many processed foods (such as cakes, biscuits and fast foods). If a food label says hydrogenated or partially hydrogenated vegetable oil then buy a different product.

With an omega 3 supplement you are looking for levels of 770mg EPA and 510mg DHA per day, and made with fish gelatine rather than bovine gelatine (see NHP's Omega 3 Support from www.naturalhealthpractice.com). If you are vegetarian then use linseed (flaxseed) oil, 1000mg per day.

Other useful nutrients

In addition to these three supplements; multivitamin and mineral, vitamin C and omega 3; there are certain specific nutrients which can be really helpful while you wean yourself off sugar and sugary foods. Many of these nutrients will be in your multivitamin and mineral but you might need extra for a short while to correct any deficiencies and get you back into good health. If you need help in putting together a good supplement programme for yourself, then do get in touch with my clinic, see *Resources* section at the back of the book.

Chromium

The nutrient that has the biggest effect on your blood sugar and control of cravings is chromium[91].

Chromium is important in general for the metabolism of carbohydrates, fats and protein but when it comes to blood sugar balance it is extremely important, as it improves the action of insulin. Chromium can help to move glucose (sugar) out of your blood, so that it can be used by your cells for energy, while also keeping the amount of glucose in your blood at a healthy level.

Chromium is found in fruits and vegetables and also whole grains but you can become deficient in chromium if you have been eating a lot of refined carbohydrates; e.g. white bread, white rice; as the chromium is lost when the grain is refined. The amount of chromium in our food will also vary depending on the richness of the soil on which the food is grown.

Foods high in added sugars like sucrose and fructose make you lose chromium via your urine so, ironically, the more of these you eat, the more deficient you become in chromium (which is, of course, the mineral you need to stop you wanting to eat these kinds of foods).

In one study, two diets were compared; one with optimal nutrients and one high in sugar. Both diets contained the same amount of chromium. The high sugar diet caused urinary chromium losses of between ten and 300 per cent. The scientists commented that 'these data demonstrate that consumption of diets high in simple sugars stimulates chromium losses'[92].

We know that people with type 2 diabetes can have low levels of chromium[93] and that when chromium is given to people with type 2 diabetes it improves blood sugar control[94].

Zinc

After chromium, zinc is the nutrient I always recommend to help control sugar cravings and blood sugar swings. Like chromium, it helps insulin to work more effectively. It can also be helpful for general appetite control, as it helps to give you a proper sense of taste and smell[95]. If you are not experiencing the full taste of your food then it is harder to appreciate the more subtle sweetness in foods, which leads you to crave and eat refined sugars to get a stronger taste.

Zinc also helps to increase the hormone leptin which controls your feelings of hunger. Leptin is the hormone that tells you when you feel satisfied and have had enough to eat. This is particularly important if you feel you always want something sweet after a meal[96].

As well as helping with blood sugar control, zinc has a widespread beneficial effect on your general health. Everyone thinks of zinc in terms of improving immune function but it is also needed for about 200 different enzyme processes in your body and for healthy cell division.

B vitamins

The B vitamins are often known as the 'stress' vitamins, as they help you cope better when you are under pressure. These vitamins are especially important if you tend to go for sugary, comfort food when you are feeling stressed.

The B vitamins are also important for efficient carbohydrate metabolism[97]. If your body doesn't use the carbohydrates you eat properly, the tendency can be to crave more carbohydrates and sugary foods.

Vitamin B1 is an important vitamin as it is needed for healthy glucose metabolism. Vitamin B6 also helps you to maintain a steady blood sugar level which helps to prevent cravings. Low levels of this vitamin have been linked to an increased risk of a number of diseases, including diabetes[98].

I have mentioned vitamin B1 and B6 in particularly but all the B vitamins are important. B2 helps to turn your food into energy, rather than being stored as fat. B3 helps to keep your blood sugar in balance and B5 is important for helping you cope with stress.

Biotin is also a member of the B vitamin family and research has shown that this nutrient is involved in blood sugar balance. A deficiency has been linked to impaired glucose tolerance and a decreased ability for your body to utilise glucose properly, resulting in higher levels of blood glucose (sugar)[99].

Vitamin D

You may just think about vitamin D in relation to bone health. However, this is another nutrient that is important in helping to keep your blood sugar in balance. Over the last few years, the amount of information about this vitamin and the numerous benefits it has in your body has exploded.

It has been found to:

- Play a major role in breast and bowel cancer prevention.

- Be important for immune function and particularly helpful in the winter, when there is more flu around.

- Help with conditions as diverse as heart disease, joint pains and arthritis, dementia, autoimmune diseases, fertility, autism and allergies.

- Help prevent or lessen SAD (seasonal affective disorder).

Unfortunately, more than half the adults in the UK have insufficient vitamin D levels[100] and we are even seeing a re-emergence of rickets in children, that was eliminated in the UK over 40 years ago.

The problem is that we are being given mixed messages over exposure to sunlight, with many experts warning us to stay covered up, or plastered in high SPF creams, because of skin cancer scares. You are most at risk in the UK of vitamin D deficiency if you do not go out much in the daytime, do not expose your skin to sunlight and if you mostly wear make-up or cosmetics with in-built sun protection factors, which you may not realise are contained in your beauty products.

The tone of your skin affects vitamin D production, so the darker your skin the more sunlight you need to produce vitamin D. Covering up large areas of skin for religious reasons will also reduce vitamin D production. It is estimated that we need about 30 minutes exposure to the sun to produce enough vitamin D. Ideally, this exposure should come from the larger areas of your body – torso and limbs - rather than purely the face.

We don't get much vitamin D from our food, as your body expects you to manufacture it through your skin from exposure to sunlight. However, some is found in oily fish, eggs and fortified breakfast cereals.

Having good levels of vitamin D is important for blood sugar balance, as it can help improve your body's sensitivity to insulin and can actually protect you against developing type 2 diabetes.

Research has shown that people who have the higher vitamin D level (greater than 62.5 nmol/l (25 ng/ml)) have a 43 per cent lower risk of developing type 2 diabetes compared to those with the lower level of vitamin D (less than 35 nmol/l (14 ng/ml))[101].

As always with nature, there is a need for balance. You shouldn't become deficient in vitamin D but equally you don't want to overload your body with it. Lately, it has become fashionable to take mega doses of vitamin D. It is a fat soluble nutrient so you can store it in your body, unlike vitamin C, which is water soluble. It can become toxic if levels become too high. If you have too low a level of vitamin D, less than 10 nmol/l (4 ng/ml) then this increases your risk of all-cause mortality (dying from any cause). But if you have a level that is too high, more than 140 nmol/l (56 ng/ml) then this also increases your risk of dying from any cause[102]. The research showed that the lowest risk of dying came with a vitamin D level of between 50-60 nmol/l but the consensus seems to be that a level between 80-100 nmol/l would be optimum.

My advice is get your vitamin D level checked. It is easy nowadays because there are simple home finger prick tests available. You will then know whether you are deficient, be given appropriate advice as to how much vitamin D you would need to take to correct that deficiency and then re-check in three months' time to make sure the level is back to normal (for a home finger blood test see www.naturalhealthpractice.com).

Vitamin E

This vitamin is known for its powerful antioxidant benefits but it is also thought to play a role in reducing the risk of developing type 2 diabetes. It improves glucose tolerance. It can also help reduce HbA1c in those people who are not controlling their blood sugar well[103]. When choosing a vitamin E supplement, look for 'd-alpha tocopherol' on the label, as this is the natural form of the vitamin. Avoid vitamin E in the form of 'dl-alpha tocopherol' as this is the synthetic version and not so easily absorbed.

Magnesium

This is an interesting mineral as it is known as 'nature's tranquiliser'. It has a very calming effect on your body generally and is helpful if you are under stress, especially if being anxious or stressed propels you to crave sugary kinds of food.

A number of studies have shown a strong association between having low levels of magnesium and type 2 diabetes[104]. In addition, higher intakes of magnesium could prevent the progression from prediabetes to full-blown diabetes[105].

Co-enzyme Q10

This is a nutrient that you produce naturally in your body. It helps with carbohydrate metabolism but, unfortunately, we produce less of it as we get older. Your cells use co-enzyme Q10 to produce energy, which is why it is often recommended in cases of fatigue.

It is a useful nutrient to reduce high blood pressure and also helps to control blood sugar[106].

Co-enzyme Q10 is a particularly important nutrient to take if you are on statins. Statins will interfere with your body's ability to produce co-enzyme Q10, resulting in lower levels in your blood. By supplementing this nutrient, it is possible to offset some of the muscle-related side effects connected with statins[107].

Also check with your doctor if you are on statins and also worried about your blood sugar because, unfortunately, statins can increase your risk of developing type 2 diabetes by almost 50 per cent[108]. Statins seem to have two negative effects on blood sugar at the same time: They decrease insulin sensitivity by 24 per cent and also reduce the pancreas' ability to secrete insulin by 12 per cent.

Alpha-lipoic acid

This nutrient is a powerful antioxidant and has been shown not only to prevent high blood pressure but also to help prevent insulin resistance[109]. It releases energy by burning glucose and, because of this, can also help with weight loss as less food is stored as fat. Research has shown that those taking alpha-lipoic acid while on a diet lost significantly more weight than those who just followed the diet[110].

L-theanine

This is an interesting amino acid that has great benefits for helping with stress. Stress is often one of the triggers for reaching for the sugary, comfort foods; so anything that can stop the cravings will be helpful. Also, as I have already explained, when your blood sugar drops stress hormones are released which can propel you to reach for that quick fix. The less your stress hormones are triggered, the calmer you will feel, the more balanced your blood sugar will be and the less you will find yourself craving sugary foods.

L-theanine can help keep you calm without causing drowsiness[111]. So it's useful when you need to feel more relaxed but also know that you need to stay sharp and focused because you have, for example, an exam or deadline. It can also help with improving concentration, attention span and learning ability.

L-theanine may also give you better quality sleep. This is very helpful if you have a tendency towards night-time snacking because of poor quality of sleep. Unlike many sleep medications (which can be addictive), l-theanine does not cause drowsiness. It helps with sleep, and especially sleep quality, by reducing anxiety, calming your mind and helping you to switch off.

We know that sleep deprivation and sleep disorders can have a serious effect on quality of life and may be the cause of many of our degenerative illnesses including heart disease and, in particular, obesity and type 2 diabetes. Sleeping badly can also lead to depression. Research has suggested that 'l-theanine is a safe natural sleep aid'[112].

In my clinic I use a supplement called Tranquil Woman Support which contains l-theanine, magnesium, B vitamins and other nutrients. Despite its name, it is also fine for men to take. See www.naturalhealthpractice.com.

CHAPTER 16

Sugar-Free Recipes

As well as reading labels and avoiding foods with added sugar, I thought you would find it useful to have some recipes that you can make at home that are healthy to eat, without added refined sugar.

Some of the recipes will have no added sweeteners in at all, other than those from the fruit, others will use natural sweeteners that I have mentioned in this book. I have tried to include a variety of sweeteners to show how they can be used.

I hope you enjoy them and you will find that as you get used to using different sweeteners that you can adapt your favourite recipes where you would have used refined sugar in the past.

With all the recipes, I recommend you try to use organic ingredients where possible, so I have not put organic eggs, organic flour, etc. throughout the recipes. With the flour I have put wholemeal, again choose organic where possible, but you can also use spelt or gluten free flour. With the oil in the recipes, you can use olive oil or experiment with other oils such as coconut.

Where you want a chocolate effect, use cacao powder which is less processed than cocoa powder. The cacao tree produces cacao pods which, when opened, contain cacao beans. It is how these beans are processed that makes the difference between cacao and cocoa. Cacao, when labelled raw, is produced by sun drying the beans and keeping the whole process below 42°C. Cocoa powder is produced using much higher temperatures so it contains less nutrients, such as antioxidants, because of the heat.

The botanical name of the tree that produces cacao and cocoa is Theobroma cacao and it is after the tree that the substance theobromine, contained in the plant, is named. It is classed as a stimulant and has a similar but lesser effect than caffeine. Theobromine can increase your heartbeat and, similar to caffeine, it can cause anxiety, restlessness and insomnia.

It is the theobromine in the chocolate which is dangerous to dogs as they metabolise this substance much more slowly than us and end up being poisoned by it.

So, I would suggest you use cacao sparingly and only when you want to serve up something a bit more special, or you know you would want to eat ordinary chocolate containing sugar and this is a better substitute.

If you would rather not have the cacao then substitute carob powder for cacao in the recipes that follow.

Some of the recipes use cup measurements and you can buy these in most kitchen supply shops or online. If you don't have the 'proper' cups then, when using dry ingredients, 1 cup is equivalent to 8oz (225g) and with liquids, 1 cup is ½ pint (237ml). The cups are relatively inexpensive to buy and make the recipes so much easier and quicker.

Tofu Fruit Whip

Serve this topped with slices of fresh fruit or on your favourite breakfast cereal.

Ingredients

100g (4oz) tofu, drained

100g (4oz) fresh or frozen fruit (strawberries, blueberries, peaches, pears, etc. (If you use some tinned fruit like mandarins then make sure the fruit is in juice rather than syrup.)

Maple syrup to taste

Dash of pure vanilla extract

1 tbsp tahini (optional)

Directions

- Blend all the ingredients until smooth. The addition of the tahini gives the whip a creamier taste.

Fig and Cranberry Balls

Ingredients

500g pack/1lb dried whole figs, hard stalk and centre of base removed, roughly chopped

85g/3oz dried apricots (buy apricots which are free from sulphur dioxide which keeps them a bright orange colour), chopped into small pieces

50g/2oz dried cranberries

100g/4oz whole almonds, lightly toasted and finely chopped

1 tbsp maple syrup optional

1 tsp ground cloves

100g/4oz sesame seeds, lightly toasted

Directions

- Put the almonds in a large bowl.
- Process the figs in a food processor until they are a smooth paste.
- Add to the almonds and then, using your hands, also mix in the dried cranberries, maple syrup and cloves.
- Roll the mixture into small balls, just to give you a mouthful.
- Put the sesame seeds onto a tray and roll the balls in them until covered.
- The balls can be eaten as they are or you can leave them on the tray to dry before eating.

Carrot and Raisin Loaf

This recipe uses liquid measures, so measure out the flour first
in a measuring jug, then the oil and then the maple syrup.
By measuring the oil before the maple syrup, you avoid the syrup sticking
to the jug. Use organic ingredients where possible.

Ingredients

125ml (4fl oz) sunflower oil

100ml (3.5fl oz) maple syrup

2 eggs

225g (8oz) carrots

100g (4oz) raisins

½ tsp baking powder

450ml (1¼ pt) wholemeal flour

½ tsp ground cinnamon

¼ tsp grated nutmeg

¼ tsp ground mixed spice

Directions

- Preheat the oven to gas mark 3/170°C/325°F. Grease a 450g (1lb) loaf tin.

- Beat the oil, maple syrup and eggs together until smooth.

- Add the carrots and raisins and combine gently.

- Fold in the baking powder, flour and spices.

- Spoon into the loaf tin and bake for 1¼ hours.

- Leave to cool before removing from the tin.

Date Slice

Ingredients

700g (1.5lbs) dates, stoned and roughly chopped

1 litre (38fl oz) porridge oats

500ml (18fl oz) wholemeal flour

175ml (6fl oz) barley malt syrup

175ml (6fl oz) sunflower oil

Directions

- Preheat the oven to 180°C/350°F. Grease a baking tin or dish 25 x 30cm (10 x 12ins).

- Place the dates in a saucepan and cover with water. Simmer until the dates are soft.

- Combine the oats and flour in a blender.

- Add the malt syrup and oil and blend thoroughly. (If you measure out the oil first and then use the same measuring jug for the barley malt, the malt just slips out easily.)

- Put three quarters of the oat mixture in the bottom of the greased tin and press it down well with your hands.

- Spread the dates over the top. Spread the remaining oat mixture on top of the dates.

- Bake for 40 minutes or until brown.

Oaty Banana Pancakes

These delicious pancakes are taken from my 12 week *Fat Around The Middle* healthy eating course and make a filling breakfast or snack.
They can be made in advance and stored in the fridge for two days.

Preparation and cooking time 25 minutes.

Ingredients

1½ cup porridge oats/gluten-free oats

1 large ripe banana, mashed with a fork

1¼ cup soya, rice or almond milk

1 egg

½ cup spelt, rice or buckwheat flour (or mix of flours)

1 tsp bicarbonate of soda

Small pinch of salt (optional)

½ tsp cinnamon (optional)

Coconut oil or ½oz butter for frying

Directions

- Put all ingredients in a jug and blend with a stick blender until smooth.

- Add 1 tsp oil and/or butter to frying pan and, when melted, add 1 tbsp of batter to the pan. Cook for a few minutes, flip and cook until underside is golden.

- Place cooked pancakes in the oven to keep them hot while you cook the rest.

- Lovely to eat on their own or with a spoon of natural yogurt with berries.

- Replace flour with more oats for a wheat-free version. Use buckwheat or rice flour for a gluten-free version.

No Added Sugar Muesli

Another recipe taken from my *Fat Around The Middle* healthy eating course.
Many mueslis found in the supermarket contain added sugars.
It's very easy to make your own at home and store it in a large jar.
One serving is 3 tbsp muesli. Serve with natural yogurt and fresh berries
for a great start to the day or a healthy snack.

Preparation time 5 minutes.

Ingredients

2 cup oat flakes

½ cup flaked almonds

½ cup walnuts

½ cup sunflower seeds

½ cup desiccated coconut

Directions

- Place ingredients in a bowl and mix well.

- For added natural sweetness add 3 tbsp unsweetened dried cranberries, unsweetened dried cherries or chopped dried apricots.

- For an even tastier version, lightly toast the muesli at 150°C for 15 minutes.

Bircher Muesli

This alternative to traditional muesli and porridge was originally created by Dr Bircher-Benner in the 1890s.

Ingredients

75mg porridge oats

25mg dried apricots or raisins

Juice from half a fresh lemon

1 apple

1 tbsp ground almonds

2 tbsp natural yogurt (cow or soya) optional

1 tbsp toasted flaked almonds

1 tsp ground cinnamon

75mg blackberries or berries of your choice

Directions

- Place the oats and dried apricots in a bowl and pour over approximately 100ml apple juice, water or oat milk and the lemon juice. Leave in the fridge for at least two hours, or overnight.

- The following morning, grate the apple and stir into the oat mix along with the ground and flaked almonds, yogurt and cinnamon.

- Transfer the muesli into bowls and top with the blackberries and a little extra sprinkled cinnamon if desired.

Fruit Jelly

It is lovely to have a fruit jelly when the weather is still warm,
but a conventional jelly is made from gelatine with colouring and sugar.
Gelatine is a protein derived from the collagen found in animal remnants,
most usually the bones.

A seaweed called agar is an easy way to make jelly.
The simplest form to use is agar powder but it can also be bought as flakes.

For a colourful jelly use red grape juice or blackcurrant (sugar-free, pure juice).

Directions

- Bring 300ml (½ pint) of juice to the boil and add 1 teaspoon of agar powder.
- Once the agar has dissolved, transfer to a dish or mould.
- The jelly can be left to set at room temperature or you can put it in the fridge.
- As it sets, add halves of seedless grapes or segments of tinned mandarin oranges (canned in fruit juice, not syrup) or berries.

Fruit and Nut Cookies

Ingredients

100g (4oz) mixed dried fruit e.g. sultanas, apricots (without mineral oil or sulphur dioxide)

200g (7oz) mixed nuts e.g. almonds, cashews, hazelnuts

1 tbsp pumpkin seeds

2 tbsp approx of sunflower seeds

75g (3oz) desiccated coconut

6 tbsp of liquid (e.g. organic apple juice, soya milk or rice milk)

Directions

- Put the dried fruit, nuts, coconut and pumpkin seeds into a food processor.

- Pulse until finely chopped and then add the liquid slowly until it makes a softish dough.

- Heap teaspoons of the dough onto a greased baking tray and press down to make rounds (5cm/2ins).

- Push some sunflower seeds into each cookie.

- Bake in a preheated over at 180°C, 350°F, gas mark 4 for about 15 minutes.

- Cool before eating.

Hazelnut Cookies Filled with Jam

Makes about 24 cookies.

Ingredients

1 cup porridge oats

1 cup hazelnuts or other nuts, like almonds, if you prefer

I cup wholemeal/spelt flour

½ tsp cinnamon

¼ tsp sea salt

½ cup oil

½ cup maple syrup

1 jar of pure fruit jam

Directions

- Pre-heat oven to 350°F/180°C.
- Lightly oil a baking tray.
- Grind the hazelnuts coarsely in a blender and put in a bowl.
- Grind the porridge oats into a flour consistency.
- Put into the same bowl as the hazelnuts and add the flour, cinnamon and salt, and combine together well.
- Whisk the oil and maple syrup together in a separate bowl.
- Add the oil/maple syrup into the dry ingredients and stir well.
- Form into small balls and press down into a 5cm (2in) round.
- Push your finger into the centre of each round to create a small hollow but without piercing the bottom.
- Put a teaspoon of jam into each hollow.
- Bake for about 15-20 minutes until lightly golden.

Date and Cacao Balls

Ingredients

12 dates, stoned

2 tbsp almond butter

2 tsp palmyra jaggery

1 tbsp flaxseeds

1 tbsp Chia seeds

1 tsp raw cacao or carob powder

1 tbsp sesame seeds

1 tbsp poppy seeds

Directions

- Put the dates in a blender and blend until they turn into a paste.
- Add the almond butter and continue to blend.
- Add the jaggery, flaxseeds, chia seeds and cacao (or carob if you prefer) until the mixture becomes dough-like.
- In a separate bowl mix the sesame seeds and poppy seeds together.
- Roll the dough into small balls and roll them in the seeds so they are completely covered.
- Put them in the fridge for 30 minutes to make the balls firm.

Lemon Icing

Ingredients

3 tbsp lemon juice

100g (4oz) tofu

1 tsp white tahini

2 tbsp maple syrup

Directions

Place all ingredients in blender and blitz until smooth.

I have put two recipes for blueberry muffins so that you can choose, as some of you may be wanting to avoid eggs or dairy.

Blueberry Muffins 1

Makes 8.

Ingredients

1½ cup wholemeal/spelt flour

½ tbsp baking powder

85g (3oz) oil

85g (3oz) rice or maple syrup

½ tsp vanilla extract

Juice and zest of one lemon

Pinch of salt

½ cup blueberries (fresh or frozen)

Directions

- Preheat oven to 325°F/170°C.
- Whisk together the wet ingredients.
- Mix together the dry ingredients.
- Combine the wet and dry ingredients and add the blueberries.
- Spoon into muffin cases.
- Cook for 25 minutes or until the centre is springy.

Blueberry Muffins 2

Makes 12.

Ingredients

110g (4oz) butter

250g (9oz) wholemeal/spelt four

250g (9oz) maple syrup

2 eggs

125ml milk/soya milk

2 tsp baking powder

Pinch of salt

225g (8oz) blueberries fresh or frozen

Directions

- Preheat oven to 350°F/180°C.
- Mix together the flour, baking powder and salt.
- In a seperate bowl, cream together the butter and maple syrup.
- Add the eggs to the butter/syrup and beat well.
- Add the milk.
- Add the dry ingredients and beat together.
- Spoon into muffin cases until about two thirds full.
- Cook for 25 minutes or until the centre is springy.

Lemon Mousse

Ingredients

¼ litre (½ pint) of water

2 tsp agar flakes

2 tbsp maple or rice syrup

¼ litre (½ pint) apple juice concentrate

1 tbsp lemon zest

2 tbsp white tahini

½ tsp vanilla extract

Directions

- Bring the water to the boil and add all the ingredients except the tahini.
- Simmer for 7-10 minutes.
- Dilute the tahini with a small amount of the simmer mixture and then add to the saucepan.
- Pour into a glass bowl and leave to set for 2-3 hours.
- Blend to a creamy consistency, you can add more water when blending if needed.

Vanilla and Lemon Pudding

Serves 4.

Ingredients

2 cup almond or soya milk

¼ cup maple syrup or ½ rice syrup

2 tbsp agar flakes or 2 tsp agar powder

2 tbsp arrowroot or cornflour

1 tsp vanilla extract

1½ lemon – juice

1½ lemon – zest

Pinch of sea salt

Directions

- Combine 1¾ cups of the milk with the maple/rice syrup and salt in a saucepan.

- Sprinkle on the agar and bring to a simmer. Only start to stir once the mixture begins to simmer. Simmer for 1 minute.

- Dissolve the arrowroot/cornflour in the remaining milk and add to the saucepan stirring quickly.

- When the mixture begins to simmer again, cook for another 1-2 minutes and then remove from the heat.

- Add in the vanilla, lemon juice and zest and pour into 4 glass sundae dishes.

- Put in fridge for about 2 hours.

This mixture can also be used as the filling for a tart, with a decoration of fruit, and berries can also be added to the almond milk before heating in the saucepan.

Crunchy Seed Bars

This recipe requires lightly toasted seeds.
You can either toast all the seeds together in a dry frying pan,
stirring all the time until they just become golden or put them on
a baking tray on a low heat in the oven.

Ingredients

1 cup lightly toasted sesame seeds

1 cup lightly toasted pumpkin seeds

1 cup lightly toasted sunflower seeds

½ cup sultanas

3-4 rice cakes, crumbled up

Barley malt syrup

Directions

- Preheat oven to 350°F/180°C.

- Brush a baking tray with oil.

- Combine all the ingredients except the barley malt into a saucepan.

- Heat the mixture and add the malt, a bit at a time, stirring with a wooden spoon.

- You want the mixture to stick on the spoon. If it does not then add more malt but do it gradually, if you add too much malt then you will lose the crunch when the mixture is cooked.

- Put the mixture onto the tray, pressing it down with the spoon to give a thickness of a bar.

- Bake for 5 minutes until golden.

- Remove from the oven, leave to cool and then cut into bars.

Corn Muffins

Makes 18.

This recipe is made with 3½ cups of wholemeal flour but if you want to introduce some healthier muffins to those who usually eat the sugar-laden ones, then change the recipe to 2½ cups of wholemeal flour and 1 cup of unbleached white flour just to make them lighter.

Ingredients

3½ cups of wholemeal/spelt flour

1 cup cornmeal

½ tsp sea salt

1½ tsp baking powder

½ cup corn oil

½ cup barley malt syrup

½ cup soya milk

2 cups apple juice

½ tbsp vanilla extract

Directions

- Preheat oven to 350°F/180°C.
- Combine all the dry ingredients in a bowl.
- Whisk or blend the wet ingredients separately.
- Add the wet ingredients to the dry and stir to mix well.
- Fill muffin cases.
- Bake for 30-40 minutes.
- Allow the muffins to cool in the tray for 5 minutes before removing.

Coconut Orange Jewels

Ingredients

1 cup desiccated coconut

1 cup walnuts

1 cup wholemeal/spelt flour

⅛ tsp sea salt

½ cup soft dates, chopped

1 tsp orange rind

½ cup orange juice

¼ cup oil

Directions

- Preheat oven to 350°F/180°C.
- Chop walnuts until they are fine.
- Add the coconut, flour and salt to the walnuts.
- Mix the wet ingredients in a blender.
- Add the wet ingredients to the dry ingredients.
- Oil a baking tray.
- Form the mixture into walnut size balls.
- Bake for 10 minutes.

Tip

If the dates are hard, then heat the orange juice, pour over the dates, soak until soft and then chop them.

Walnut and Lemon Bread

This can be made as a loaf or spooned into muffin cases (makes 24 muffins).

Ingredients

½ cup of walnuts

½ cup of apple juice

¼ cup of lemon juice

½ cup of oil

½ cup of maple syrup

2 cups of wholemeal flour/spelt

Grated peel of two lemons (better to get them unwaxed)

2 tsp baking powder

Pinch of sea salt

Directions

- Preheat oven to 375°F/190°C.
- Lightly roast and then chop the walnuts.
- Blend together the lemon juice, rind, apple juice, oil and maple syrup.
- In a bowl combine together the flour, baking powder and salt.
- Add the wet ingredients to the dry and mix to a smooth batter.
- Fold in the walnuts.
- Pour into muffin cases or an oiled loaf tin.
- Bake for 15 minutes.
- Reduce the heat to 350°F/180°C and cook for another 20 minutes.

These next recipes are from Helen Ford, one of my senior nutritionists, who has been working with me for over 11 years.

Protein Powerballs

Makes 30 – 40.

Preparation time 25 mins.

Ingredients

1 cup peanut/almond/hazelnut butter

2½ cup shelled hempseeds (or milled flaxseeds if not available)

1 tbsp carob powder

½ cup nuts (any combination of peanuts, sliced almonds, chopped walnuts, chopped cashews, toasted coconut)

½ cup dried fruit (raisins, sultanas, cranberries, chopped apricots, chopped dates)

Directions

- Mix all the ingredients together until well combined. If mix is too dry add more nut butter.

- Roll into small balls and eat!

- Keep dipping hands in bowl of clean water to prevent mixture from sticking.

- Can be rolled in finely chopped nuts and seeds.

- Can be frozen, with greaseproof paper separating the layers, for up to one month.

Nut Cookies
Makes 12.

Ingredients

200g mixed nuts (walnuts, almonds, pecans, hazelnuts)

100g mixed dried fruit (prunes, apricots, sultanas)

1 tbsp pumpkin seeds

75g desiccated coconut or ground almonds

6 tbsp soya/rice/oat milk

1 to 2 tbsp sunflower seeds

Directions

- Put the nuts, fruit, pumpkin seeds and coconut or almonds into a food processor.
- Pulse until finely chopped, then gradually add the soya/oat/rice milk until you have a softish dough.
- Place heaped teaspoons on a baking tray and press down with a spoon to a 5cm (2in) round.
- Sprinkle over the seeds and push them into the dough.
- Bake in a preheated oven at 350°F/180°C, gas mark 4 for 15 minutes or until lightly browned.
- Cool for 5 minutes on the tray, then store in sealed container.

Tip

Vanilla or almond essence can be added for a different taste.

Try ground cinnamon and/or ginger to give an extra bite!

Nutty Protein Balls

Ingredients

1 cup raw, whole almonds

1 cup of Medjool or soft dates

1 tbsp almond or cashew butter

3 tbsp coconut oil

3 tbsp carob or raw cacao powder

2 tsp ground cinnamon

1 tsp maple syrup

Directions

- Put the almonds in the food processor and blitz until crumb consistency.

- Add the rest of the ingredients and process until well combined.

- Using damp hands roll the mixture into balls and place in fridge.

Coconut Flour Banana Bread

Ingredients

4 eggs

¾ cup mashed banana (2-3 fresh or frozen bananas)

¼ cup coconut oil, melted

¼ cup coconut milk

2 tbsp maple syrup

½ tsp pure vanilla extract

¼ tsp ground ginger

½ cup coconut flour

½ tsp baking powder

Directions

- Preheat oven to 350°F/180°C and line an 8 x 4 inch loaf tin with parchment paper across both sides for easy lifting. Set aside.

- Combine eggs, bananas, coconut milk, oil, maple syrup, vanilla extract and ginger in a large bowl with an electric mixer (using a mixer gives this bread an airier texture than mixing by hand).

- Whisk coconut flour and baking powder in a small bowl. Once mixed, slowly add the dry ingredients to the wet mixture and mix until smooth.

- Pour batter into prepared loaf tin and bake in preheated oven for 40-45 minutes or until skewer inserted comes out clean.

- Remove from the oven and allow to cool for five minutes. Remove from pan and allow to cool on a cooling rack for 20-40 minutes before slicing and serving.

I would like to thank Heather Leeson, my senior nutritionist in Ireland, for these next recipes.

Apple Fruit Cake

Preparation and baking time 75 minutes.

Ingredients

125ml olive oil or melted butter or coconut oil (allow to cool before using)

1 tsp vanilla extract or vanilla powder

¼ cup maple syrup

3 free range eggs

280g wholemeal spelt flour

2 tbsp ground flaxseeds

Pinch sea salt

1 tsp ground cinnamon

1 tsp baking powder

80g raisins

80g apricots, chopped into small pieces

Zest and juice of one orange

2 apples (250g) finely chopped. No need to peel

Directions

- Preheat oven to 160°C.

- Mix together the oil/butter, vanilla, maple syrup and eggs.

- Place flour, flax seeds, salt, cinnamon, baking powder, orange zest and juice and dried fruit in a large bowl and mix well. Then pour in the oil mixture and stir well.

- Add the apple pieces and gently combine, then place mixture in a loaf tin lined with greaseproof paper and bake for one hour or until a skewer comes out clean when inserted.

- Allow to cool completely in the tin before removing and serving.

For a higher protein version, replace 100g of the flour with ground almonds. You may need to adjust the amount of orange juice you add too.

Chocolate Peanut Butter Cookies

Preparation and baking time 15 minutes.

Ingredients

1 cup unsweetened peanut butter

1 tbsp raw cacao or carob powder

1 tbsp chia seeds

1 large egg

½ tbsp maple or brown rice syrup

Directions

- Preheat oven to 180°C and line a baking sheet with greaseproof paper.

- Add all ingredients to a bowl and mix well. This can also be done in a food processor.

- Roll the dough into balls, place on the baking sheet and flatten with your hand or a fork.

- Bake for 8-10 minutes and allow to cool before eating.

- Best eaten within 24 hours.

Gingerbread Cookies

Preparation and baking time 45 minutes.

Ingredients

280g finely ground wholemeal spelt flour/wholemeal flour

½ tsp baking powder

1 tsp ground cinnamon

¼ tsp ground nutmeg

¼-½ tsp ground ginger

120g soft pitted dates e.g. Medjool

100ml olive oil/softened butter

120g maple syrup

1 tsp vanilla extract

1 egg white

Directions

- Blend flour, baking powder, spices and dates in a food processor until mixture is crumbly.

- Add oil, maple syrup, vanilla extract and egg white and process until a soft dough forms.

- Place the dough between 2 pieces of greaseproof paper and press with hand or rolling pin until less than ½ cm thick. Then place dough in the fridge for 1 hour or in the freezer for 20 minutes to firm up.

- Preheat oven to 150°C.

- Cut out shapes, place on tray lined with greaseproof paper and bake for about 30 minutes or until golden.

- Allow to cool completely before eating.

Coconut and Banana Bread

This is another recipe for a coconut bread,
but the ingredients are slightly different.

Preparation and cooking time 75 minutes.

Ingredients

400g ripe bananas*

6 eggs

6-8 pitted dates (use Medjool dates where possible, or pre-soak drier dates in a little hot water for a couple of hours before using, to soften)

3 tbsp coconut oil, butter or olive oil

1 tsp vanilla powder/extract

1 tsp cinnamon

2 tsp baking powder

70g coconut flour

20g ground linseeds

Directions

- Preheat oven to 170°C and line and lightly oil a bread tin.

- In a food processor, blend the bananas, eggs, dates, coconut oil.

- Place the dry ingredients in a mixing bowl and stir, then add in the banana mixture and stir well until combined.

- Pour into bread tin, smooth the top and scatter with shredded coconut.

- Leave for 10 minutes and then bake for 50-60 minutes until firm to the touch.

- Allow to cool in the tin before turning out.

- Will keep in the fridge for up to one week and can also be frozen. Perfect for lunchboxes, just add a frozen slice in the morning, will be defrosted by break time.

Tip: *Peel, quarter and freeze ripe bananas to use in baking and in smoothies. Just allow to defrost partially before using in this recipe.*

Chocolate Cranberry Bites

Preparation time 10 minutes.

Ingredients

1 cup pecans or use a mix of walnuts, cashews, hazelnuts

1½ tbsp raw cacao or carob powder

¾ cup soft pitted dates

1 tsp vanilla extract

1 tbsp ground linseeds/shelled hemp seeds

2 tbsp dried cranberries (or quantity as desired)

Directions

- Blitz nuts and cacao powder in a food processor until coarsely ground.

- Add dates, vanilla extract and linseeds/hemp seeds and blend until smooth.

- Add cranberries and pulse briefly.

- Press the mixture firmly into a plastic container and freeze for 1 hour to set. Store in the fridge (will keep for up to 2 weeks) or in the freezer (will keep for up to 2 months).

Apricot Cashew Nut Bites

Ingredients

1 cup cashew nuts (or pecans, walnuts or other nuts or seeds)

Pinch sea salt

½ cup dried apricots

½ cup Medjool or other soft dates (pitted)

1 large tbsp almond butter (or hazelnut, peanut or other nut butter)

½ cup shelled hemp seeds/sesame seeds

½ tsp cinnamon (or replace with vanilla or other spices)

Directions

- Place the nuts in a food processor and blend until coarsely ground.
- Add remainder of ingredients and blend until dried fruit is well chopped and mixture holds together when pressed. Add a tiny splash of water if too dry.
- Roll mixture into small balls and store in an airtight container in the fridge (will keep for up to 2 weeks) or in the freezer (will keep for up to 2 months).

Tropical Ice Lollies

Preparation time 10 minutes.

Ingredients

2 ripe peaches, quartered and stoned or ½ ripe pineapple, cored and roughly chopped

100ml tinned unsweetened coconut milk (chose one with at least 98 per cent coconut)

½ tsp vanilla extract (with peaches) or small knob fresh ginger, grated (with pineapple)

Directions

- Place ingredients in a blender until smooth.
- Pour into 4 ice lolly moulds and freeze for at least 3 hours.

You can replace the peaches with 2 handfuls of berries or other fruit of your choice.

Coconut Yogurt

Many commercial dairy and soya yogurts contain sugar or sugar substitutes. This recipe, adapted from one by Irish food writer Susan Jane White, needs only five ingredients and a large jar.

It tastes great served with fruit or instead of cream or custard.

Ingredients

1 block/200g creamed coconut

300ml hot filtered water

1 capsule of a good quality probiotic e.g. NHP's Advanced Probiotic Support

½ tsp vanilla powder or cinnamon

1 tsp maple syrup/brown rice syrup

Directions

- Roughly chop the coconut cream, then place in a food processor with the hot water and blend until completely smooth.

- Leave to cool (must be no warmer than luke warm) then add the contents of the probiotic capsule (just pull the capsule apart and use the contents), vanilla and sweetener. The sweetener is not essential, but provides food for the beneficial bacteria to ferment the yogurt.

- Pour mixture into a very clean kilner jar, large jam jar or other glass container and cover with kitchen paper and an elastic band.

- Keep in a warm place e.g. on a kitchen counter or airing cupboard. After 12 hours, stir the mixture thoroughly with a plastic fork. This will prevent the yogurt splitting. Leave for a further 1 to 2 days before tasting and refrigerating. The yogurt will continue to thicken over the next few days.

Berry Frozen Yogurt

Preparation time 5 minutes.

Ingredients

300g frozen berries

4-6 tbsp natural yogurt

1 tbsp maple syrup (optional)

Directions

- Place ingredients in a food processor and blend until smooth.

- Serve immediately.

- Store in the freezer for up to 2 months. Remove from freezer 20 minutes before serving to allow to soften slightly.

Chia Jam

Most jams contain at least 50 per cent sugar. For a quick and healthier version, try making this simple chia jam using fresh seasonal fruit or even frozen fruit.

Preparation and cooking time 15 minutes.

Ingredients

2 cups fruit e.g. nectarines, berries

1½ tbsp chia seeds

½ tbsp maple syrup (optional, should not be needed with ripe fruit)

Directions

- Heat fruit in a saucepan for around 10 minutes, breaking it up as it cooks until no chunks remain.

- Add chia seeds and stir well to combine.

- Taste and add maple syrup if necessary.

- Place in a glass jar with a lid and store in the fridge for up to 7 days. Will thicken as it cools.

Healthier 'Chocolate Spread'

Preparation time 5 minutes.

Ingredients:

½ jar hazelnut butter

3 large medjool dates, pitted

1½ tbsp raw cacao powder

1 tsp vanilla extract or vanilla bean paste

Directions:

- Blitz ingredients in a food processor until smooth.
- Store in the fridge for up to 1 week.

Healthy Flapjacks

Preparation and baking time 40 minutes.

Ingredients

1 cup soft pitted dates

½ cup brown rice syrup

¾ cup coconut oil or butter, melted

1 cup ground almonds

2 cup oats

½ cup walnuts, pecans or almonds, roughly broken

Handful of sunflower seeds

½ cup raisins

1 tsp cinnamon

Directions

- Preheat oven to 170°C.

- Using a hand blender or food processor roughly blend brown rice syrup, melted oil / butter and dates.

- Mix other ingredients together in a bowl, add the date mixture and combine well.

- Scrape into a flapjack tin pre-lined with grease proof paper, smooth and bake for approx 30 minutes or until golden.

- Leave in the tin, allow to cool and then place in fridge for at least three hours before cutting and eating.

- Will keep in the fridge for up to 2 weeks.

Based on a recipe from Irish food writer Susan Jane White.

**Here are some savoury recipes from Heather Leeson,
as many of the savoury foods on the market are sugar-laden.**

Many cooking sauces contain added sugar or sugar substitutes.
It is much healthier and cheaper to make your own versions.

Stir-Fry Sauce

Preparation time 10 minutes.

Ingredients

2 tbsp soy sauce

½ tbsp rice wine like mirin or sherry wine

½ tbsp sesame seed oil

2cm fresh ginger, finely minced or grated

2 cloves garlic, finely minced or grated

Fresh chilli, finely chopped (optional)

Directions

- Mix all ingredients together in screw top jar. Use 1 tbsp per stir-fry portion. Store in fridge for up to 1 week.

Asian-Style Salad Dressing

Preparation time 10 minutes.

Ingredients

Small piece fresh ginger, grated

Juice of 2 limes

1 tbsp soy sauce

1 tbsp sesame seed oil (optional)

150ml olive oil

Directions

- Place ingredients in a screw top jar and shake well to mix.

- Will keep in the fridge for up to 3 days. Shake before use.

Red Pesto

Preparation time 10 minutes.

Ingredients

1½ cups sundried tomatoes in oil

½ cup chopped almonds

1½ cups olive oil (use oil that tomatoes were stored in)

1 clove garlic, crushed or grated (optional)

2 handfuls fresh basil

1 tbsp balsamic vinegar

½ tsp cayenne pepper

Directions

- Blend sundried tomatoes and almonds in food processor for a minute or two.

- Then add in remaining ingredients and blend until desired consistency achieved.

- This will keep in the fridge for up to 2 weeks. Store in a jam jar or other air tight container and ensure that the pesto is covered with a thin layer of olive oil.

Ways to use red pesto

- Mix 1 tbsp pesto with 3 tbsp full fat natural yogurt to make a healthy dip. Perfect for parties and lunchboxes.

- Toss pesto through some wholegrain pasta and serve with a green salad.

- Crunchy pesto cod - mix pesto with wholemeal breadcrumbs and use to top white fish e.g. cod. Bake in oven and serve with steamed vegetables.

- Pesto pizza - spread 2 tsp pesto on a wholegrain wrap, top with veg and mozzarella/feta and bake for 6-8 minutes.

- Use as marinade for grilled prawns or fish.

- Spread a wholegrain toasted pitta bread with ½ tbsp red pesto. Fill the pitta with green salad and a little soft goat's cheese.

Simple Tomato and Red Pepper Sauce

Preparation and cooking time 30 minutes.

You may be surprised to learn that many commercial brands
of tomato sauce contain added sugar.
Check the labels of the products you buy or try this simple recipe.
Extra sauce can be frozen to be used later or kept in the fridge for 4 days.

Ingredients

½ jar roasted peppers (stored in olive oil), drained

2 tbsp olive oil (or use the oil from the peppers)

1 large/2 small red onions, finely chopped

2 cloves garlic, crushed

2 tins organic whole plum tomatoes, sugar free

Salt and pepper

Directions

- Gently fry the onions and garlic in the olive oil over a low heat for 6 minutes or until softening.

- Add in the tomatoes and peppers and simmer uncovered over a low heat for 20 minutes.

- Blend with a stick blender and season to taste.

- For extra protein and to make a more filling sauce add a cup of red lentils with the tomatoes and peppers.

- For a more traditional Italian tomato sauce omit the peppers and add a handful of fresh basil when blending.

Use this sauce as a base for cooking white fish. Simply place the sauce in a
pan, top with a fillet of fish, cover and simmer gently for 10 – 14 minutes or
until fish is cooked.

It can also be used as a base for a soup. Just thin with 750ml water and
2 tsp vegetable bouillon for tomato and red pepper soup.

Healthy Teriyaki Sauce

Preparation time 10 minutes.

Ingredients

¾ cup mirin, rice wine

1 cup soy sauce

4 tbsp lime juice

3 tsp ground ginger/thumb size piece fresh ginger, grated

1 clove garlic, grated

1 tbsp sesame seeds, lightly toasted

2 spring onions, finely sliced

Directions

- Place mirin, soya sauce, lime juice, ginger and garlic in a saucepan. Bring to the boil and simmer gently for 5 minutes.
- When serving, top with sesame seeds and spring onions.
- Store in the fridge for up to 3 days.

For Teriyaki salmon, poach salmon fillets in Teriyaki sauce in covered pan over medium heat for 8 – 12 minutes, depending on thickness of fillet. Serve with stir-fried vegetables and brown rice.

Spiced Seeds

Preparation and cooking time 30 minutes.

Ingredients

1 tsp coconut oil

250g mixed seeds (pumpkin, sunflower, sesame, linseed)

½-1 tsp smoked paprika

½-1 tsp cinnamon

2 tsp tamari

1-2 tsp maple syrup

Directions

- Preheat oven to 160°C and line a baking sheet with greaseproof paper.

- Mix all ingredients together in a bowl and spread onto baking sheet. Cook for 15-20 minutes until golden. Stir once or twice during cooking.

- Allow to cool and store in an airtight container. Use as a snack or to liven up salads or scatter on top of soups.

- Try using 1 tsp mixed spice, 1 tsp cinnamon and ½ tsp cayenne pepper with an extra teaspoon maple syrup for a sweeter version. Or use curry powder or other spice blend for a different flavour.

Conclusion

Knowledge really is power. So many people have absolutely no idea just how dangerous sugar is to their health. They simply don't realise that, by consuming sugar on a regular and excessive basis, they are putting themselves at risk of a host of chronic diseases such as type 2 diabetes, cancer, heart disease and dementia. They simply haven't realised the link between a high-sugar diet and weight gain, stress and premature ageing.

The food manufacturers, advertisers, supermarkets and government haven't helped either. The aisles are laden with sugar-saturated products and television is infected with advertisements for these products, often targeting children who already have a naturally sweet tooth.

It's not easy cutting down on sugar under these circumstances but I hope that, having read this book, you now understand exactly what sugar is (in its myriad forms) and why it is so important that you try to reduce it in your diet.

You may decide that you will reduce sugar gradually; buying different brands of foods as you run out e.g. swapping your usual jam for a pure fruit, no sugar one and trying some of the alternative natural sweeteners mentioned in this book. But you may prefer to go for the five day sugar detox and then for the future keep out all the added sugary foods and drinks except on social occasions when a piece of birthday cake is fine.

As you reduce sugar in your diet, you will inevitably notice improvements in various areas of your health and in life in general. You will find that balancing your blood sugar naturally will give you far more sustained energy – it's very likely that you won't experience those horrible mid-morning or mid-afternoon energy slumps, the ones that lead you to reach for the cookies or chocolate. Your weight will naturally start to regulate itself and your sleep patterns will improve.

Those kinds of benefits can motivate you to continue removing sugar from your life, watching out for sugar in the labels on the food you buy and re-educating your taste buds so you no longer crave extreme sweet tastes. Remember just how addictive sugar is – you very probably have a serious sugar addiction so be gentle on yourself as you start on your journey to a healthy, sugar-free or 'sugar-less' you.

One of the huge rewards of going sugar-free is that you rediscover the pleasure in 'normal' food – when your taste-buds are no longer habituated to sugar, they will find the simplest of foods sweet and delicious. A simple apple can be a revelation. Peas and carrots will taste like nectar. Even water can taste sweet when it's not being compared to soft drinks full of sugar or artificial sweeteners.

I recommend that you re-read this book from time-to-time, to remind yourself of why you are adjusting your eating and drinking habits. You might also want to share it with your partner, family and friends so they understand why you're changing your eating habits. Also, I have found that if you substitute a sugar-free jam, tomato ketchup or mayonnaise, everyone else eats them as they can't tell the difference. Explore the recipes together and experiment with sugar-free cooking. When I started out in nutrition, over 30 years ago, there was very little choice in the supermarkets. Nowadays there are a host of natural and sugar-free products to help you make the transition. You can have sweet foods that are not laden with either sugar or unpleasant artificial sweeteners. There are also so many resources online now too – you need never be at a loss when it comes to finding a substitute for your favourite foods and ways of adapting your favourite recipes.

My top ten tips to help you go sugar-free

- Become label-aware. Take the time to read labels in the shops and avoid products that contain refined sugar.

- Eat little and often to balance your blood sugar levels.

- Have three good protein-based meals a day plus snacks (including protein) mid-morning and mid-afternoon.

- Try to cut down on caffeine – it can cause a drop in blood sugar that can trigger sugar cravings.

- Add protein to carbohydrate meals and snacks to slow down the (natural) sugar release.

- When you feel yourself craving something sweet, pause and ask yourself what emotion you're feeling and what you really need.

- Drink plenty of water. Often we feel hungry when actually we're dehydrated.

- Chew your food really well and eat slowly.

- Do try the recipes in this book. Realising that you can avoid sugar and yet still eat a wide variety of delicious foods will be reassuring. Life without sugar doesn't mean the end of good eating!

- Remember the 80/20 rule – the occasional piece of chocolate cake is no big deal. It's what you're eating on a daily basis that counts.

Do consider supplements. I really feel that these days we can all use good supplementation. So, remember those bedrocks of good nutrition – a good quality multivitamin and mineral, backed up by vitamin C and omega 3 essential fatty acids. The multi should contain good levels of the B vitamins, chromium, magnesium, vitamins D and E and other nutrients to help balance your blood sugar, stave off cravings and give you a real boost of vitality.

Coming off sugar entirely is a life-changing step which creates huge rewards, not just in the short term but for your long term health and longevity. I do appreciate that losing sugar from your life can be hard – it's a tough, dramatic change – but I promise you will be surprised at how quickly your health will improve.

I know from years of working with patients in the clinic that going sugar-free really can have a huge effect. I promise you that my methods do work. This book will have armed you with the tools you need to make informed decisions about your health, and to recognise exactly how much sugar (obvious and hidden) you may be eating in your diet. My sincere hope is that it will inspire you to take a big step towards a healthy, happy, truly sweet life – without sugar!

Never forget, your life and your health lies in your hands.

Wishing you the best of health,

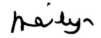

Resources

Glenville Nutrition Clinics
Natural Healthcare for Women

CONSULTATIONS:

If you would like to have a consultation (either in person, on the telephone or by Skype), then please feel free to phone my clinic for an appointment.

All the qualified nutritionists who work in my UK and Irish clinics have been trained by me in my specific approach to nutrition and women's healthcare.

THE CLINICS ARE LOCATED IN:

UK - Harley Street, London and Tunbridge Wells, Kent.

To book a personal or telephone appointment at any of these clinics, or for more information, please contact us at:

Glenville Nutrition Clinic
14 St John's Road,
Tunbridge Wells,
Kent, TN4 9NP.

Tel: 01892 515905
Int. Tel: +44 1 892 515905
Email: health@marilynglenville.com
Website: www.marilynglenville.com

Ireland - Dublin, Galway and Cork

To book a personal or telephone appointment at any of these clinics, or for more information, please contact us at:

Tel: 01 402 0777 | **Website:** www.glenvillenutrition.ie

Talks and Seminars: I frequently give talks and seminars. See my website for my upcoming schedule, under Events: www.marilynglenville.com. If you would like to organise a talk near you, I would be happy to come and speak - call my clinic and ask for information about how to arrange this.

Supplements and Tests: The Natural Health Practice (NHP) is my supplier of choice for all the supplements and tests mentioned in this book. They only carry products that I use in my clinics and are in the correct form, the right amounts and use the highest quality ingredients. For more information, please contact:

Website: www.naturalhealthpractice.com
Tel: 0845 8800915 | **Int. Tel:** + 44 1 892 507598

IF YOU HAVE ENJOYED THIS BOOK THEN PLEASE SEND A REVIEW.

I also invite you to join me on Facebook and Twitter for more information, tips and updates on my work.

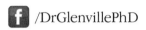 /DrGlenvillePhD

@DrGlenville

FREE HEALTH TIPS

If you would like to receive my exclusive Health Tips by email, drop me a line at health@marilynglenville.com. Just mention "Free Health Tips" in the subject line and you will be added to my special list to receive regular health tips and other useful information.

OTHER BOOKS BY DR MARILYN GLENVILLE PHD

Fat Around the Middle – How to Lose that Bulge for Good

Getting Pregnant Faster

Natural Solutions to the Menopause

Healthy Eating for the Menopause Cookbook

Natural Solutions to PCOS

Natural Solutions to IBS

The Natural Health Bible for Women

Osteoporosis – How to Prevent, Treat and Reverse

The Nutritional Health Handbook for Women

Overcoming PMS The Natural Way

RECIPES

If you have any sugar-free recipes you would like to share and especially if you've used any of the alternative sweeteners suggested in this book, please send them to me health@marilynglenville.com stating the subject: Sugar-free recipe and I will include them on my website and, if I get enough, put them in a sugar-free cookbook and mention your name.

References

Chapter 1

Page 11   1 Welsh JA et al, 2010, Caloric sweetener consumption and dyslipidemia among US adults, *JAMA*, 303, 15, 1490-7

Chapter 2

Page 17   2 Nickerson KP et al, 2014, The dietary polysaccharide maltodextrin promotes Salmonella survival and mucosal colonization in mice, *PLoS One*, 9, 7

Chapter 3

Page 18   3 http://www.nutrition.org.uk/attachments/article/190/763_BNF%20 Annual%20Report%202013-14.pdf

Page 20   4 Bello NT et al, 2011, Opioidergic consequences of dietary-induced binge eating, *Physiology and Behavior*, 104, 1, 98-104.

5 Lenoir M, Serre F, Cantin L, Ahmed SH (2007) Intense Sweetness Surpasses Cocaine Reward. *PLoS ONE* 2(8): e698. doi:10.1371/journal.pone.0000698

Page 21   6 Lennerz B et al, 2013, Effects of dietary glycemic index on brain regions related to reward and craving in men, *Am J Clin Nutr*, 98, 3, 641-647

Page 23   7 Teff KL et al, 2009, Endocrine and metabolic effects of consuming fructose- and glucose-sweetened beverages with meals in obese men and women: influence of insulin resistance on plasma triglyceride responses, *J Clin Endocrinol Metab*, 94, 5, 1562-9

Chapter 4

Page 25   8 Donga E et al, 2010, A single night of partial sleep deprivation induces insulin resistance in multiple metabolic pathways in healthy subjects, *J Clin Endocrinol Metab*, 95, 6 , 2963-8

9 Spiegel K et al (1999), Impact of sleep debt on metabolic and endocrine function, *Lancet*, 354, 1435-39)

Page 28   10 Just T et al, 2008, Cephalic phase insulin release in healthy humans after taste stimulation? *Appetite*, 51, 3, 622-7

Chapter 5

Page 29   11 Finking G, Hanke H, 1997, Nikolaj Nikolajewitsch Anitschkow (1885-1964) established the cholesterol-fed rabbit as a model for atherosclerosis research, *Atherosclerosis*, 135, 1, 1-7

12 Keys A, 1970, Coronary heart disease in seven countries. I. The study program and objectives. *Circulation,* 41, (4 Suppl) I1-8 and Keys A, 1970, Coronary heart disease in seven countries. Summary. *Circulation*, 41, (4 Suppl), I186-95

Page 30   13 Benatar JR et al, 2014, A randomised trial evaluating the effects of change in dairy food consumption on cardio-metabolic risk factors, *Eur J Prev Cardiol*, 21, 11, 1376-86

14 Harcombe Z et al, 2015, Evidence from randomised controlled trials did not support the introduction of dietary fat guidelines in 1977 and 1983: a systematic review and meta-analysis, *BMJ Open Heart*, 2: doi:10.1136/openhrt-2014-000196

Page 31   15 Johnson RK et al, 2009, Dietary Sugars Intake and Cardiovascular Health: A Scientific Statement From the American Heart Association, *Circulation*, 120, 1011-1020

Page 32   16 Setola E et al, 2004, Insulin resistance and endothelial function are improved after folate and vitamin B12 therapy in patients with metabolic syndrome: relationship between homocysteine levels and hyperinsulinemia, *Eur J Endocrinol*, 15, 4, 483-9

17 Mayor S, Statins associated with 46% rise in type 2 diabetes risk, study shows. *BMJ*, 2015, doi: 10.1136/bmj.h1222.

18 Besseling J et al, 2015, Association between familial hypercholesterolemia and prevalence of type 2 diabetes mellitus, *JAMA*, 313, 10, 1029-36

19 Henriksbo BD et al, 2014, Fluvastatin causes NLRP3 inflammasome-mediated adipose insulin resistance. *Diabetes*, 63, 11, 3742-7

Page 33   20 Ulmer H et al, 2004, Why Eve Is Not Adam: Prospective Follow-Up in 149,650 Women and Men of Cholesterol and Other Risk Factors Related to Cardiovascular and All-Cause Mortality, *Journal of Women's Health*, 13, 1, 41-53

21 Walsh JME, Pignone, 2004, Drug treatment of hyperlipidemia in women, *JAMA*, 291, 2243-52

22 Hodis HN, Mack WJ, 2007, Postmenopausal hormone therapy in clinical perspective, *Menopause*, 14, 1-14

23 Sachdeva A et al, 2009, Lipid levels in patients hospitalized with coronary artery disease: an analysis of 136,905 hospitalizations in Get With the Guidelines. *Am Heart J*, 57:111-1170

24 Al-Mallah MH et al, 2009, Low admission LDL-cholesterol is associated with increased 3-year all-cause mortality in patients with non ST segment elevation myocardial infarction. *Cardiol J*, 16, 227-33

25 L Godfrey et al, 2014, Arginine-directed glycation and decreased HDL plasma concentration and functionality, *Nutrition & Diabetes*, 4, e134

Chapter 6

Page 34   26 Ma RC et al, 2014, Causes of type 2 diabetes in China, *Lancet Diabetes Endocrinol*, 2, 12, 980-91

Page 34   27 Mainous AG et al, 2014, Prevalence of prediabetes in England from 2003 to 2011: population-based, cross-sectional study. *BMJ Open*, 4, 6

Page 36   28 http://blog.fooducate.com//2010/08/01/ada-response-to-accusations-on-partnership-with-hershey/

Page 37   29 de la Monte SM et al, 2012, Dysfunctional Pro-Ceramide, ER Stress, and Insulin/IGF Signaling Networks with Progression of Alzheimer's Disease. *J Alzheimer's Dis*, 30, S217-229

Page 38   30 Basu S et al, 2013, The Relationship of Sugar to Population-Level Diabetes Prevalence: An Econometric Analysis of Repeated Cross-Sectional Data. *PLoS ONE* 8(2): e57873

           31 Romaquera D, 2013, Consumption of sweet beverages and type 2 diabetes incidence in European adults: results from EPIC-InterAct, *Diabetologia*, 56, 7, 1520-30

           32 Fagherazzi G et al, 2013, Consumption of artificially and sugar-sweetened beverages and incident type 2 diabetes in the Etude Epidémiologique auprès des femmes de la Mutuelle Générale de l'Education Nationale–European Prospective Investigation into Cancer and Nutrition cohort, *Am J Clin Nutr*, 97, 3, 571-23

Page 39   33 Habib SL, Rojna, 2013, Diabetes and risk of Cancer, *Oncol*, 583786

           34 De Beer JC, Liebenberg, 2014, Does cancer risk increase with HbA1c, independent of diabetes? *Br J Cancer*, 110, 9, 2361-8

Chapter 7

Page 41   35 McNay E, presented at the Annual Society for Neuroscience meeting in San Diego, USA, December 2013

Page 42   36 De la Monte S and Wands JR, 2005, Review of insulin and insulin-like growth factor expression, signaling and malfunction in the central nervous system: Relevance to Alzheimer's disease, *Journal of Alzheimer's Disease*, 7, 1, 45-61

           37 Bitel CL et al, 2012, Amyloid-β and tau pathology of Alzheimer's disease induced by diabetes in a rabbit animal model. *J Alzheimers Dis*, 32, 2, 291-305

Page 43   38 Talbot, K et al, 2012, Demonstrated brain insulin resistance in Alzheimer's disease patients is associated with IGF-1 resistance, IRS-1 dysregulation, and cognitive decline. *J. Clin. Invest.* 122, 1316– 1338

           39 Bayer-Carter JL et al, 2011, Diet intervention and cerebrospinal fluid biomarkers in amnestic mild cognitive impairment. *Arch Neurol*, 68, 6, 743-52

           40 Crane PK et al, 2013, Glucose levels and risk of dementia, *Eng J Med*, 369, 6, 540-8

Page 44   41 Volicer L et al, 2001, Sundowning and circadian rhythms in Alzheimer's disease. *Am J Psychiatry*, 158, 5, 704-11

42 Kang JE et al, 2009, Amyloid-beta dynamics are regulated by orexin and the sleep-wake cycle. *Science*, 326, 5955, 1005-7

Chapter 8

Page 45   43 Giovannucci E, 2005, The role of insulin resistance and hyperinsulinemia in cancer causation. *Curr Med Chem*, 5, 1, 53-60)

44 Warburg O, 1956, On the origin of cancer cells. *Science*, 123, 309-14.

Page 46   45 Silver SA et al, 2005, Dietary carbohydrates and breast cancer risk: a prospective study of the roles of overall glycemic index and glycemic load, *Int J Cancer*, 114, 4, 653-8

46 Stocks T et al, 2009, Blood glucose and risk of incident and fatal cancer in the metabolic syndrome and cancer project (me-can): analysis of six prospective cohorts. *PLoS Med* 6, 12

47 Kabat et al, 2009, Repeated measures of serum glucose and insulin in relation to postmenopausal breast cancer. *Int J Cancer*, 125, 11, 2704-10

48 Walker-Samuel S et al, 2013, In vivo imaging of glucose uptake and metabolism in tumors. *Nat Med*, 19, 1067-1072

Page 47   49 Krone CA, Ely JT, 2005, Controlling hyperglycemia as an adjunct to cancer therapy. *Integr Cancer Ther*, 4, 1, 25-31

Chapter 9

Page 49   50 Shiloah E et al, 2003, Effect of Acute Psychotic Stress in Nondiabetic Subjects on β-Cell Function and Insulin Sensitivity, *Diabetes Care*, 26, 5, 1462-1467

51 Yun AJ, Doux JD, 2007, Unhappy meal: how our need to detect stress may have shaped our preferences for taste, *Med Hypotheses*, 69, 4, 746-5

52 Zellner DA et al, 2006, Food selection changes under stress, *Physiol Behav*, 87, 4, 789-93

Page 50   53 Do Vale S et al, 2014, The relationship between dehydroepiandrosterone (DHEA), working memory and distraction--a behavioral and electrophysiological approach. *PLoS One*, 9, 8, e104869

Chapter 10

Page 53   54 Noordam R et al, 2011, High serum glucose levels are associated with a higher perceived age, *Age*, 35, 1, 189-95

55 Gkogkolou P, Bohm M, Advanced glycation end products: Key players in skin aging?, *Dermatoendocrinol*, 4, 3, 259-70

Page 54   56 Fitzpatrick AL et al, 2007, Leukocyte telomere length and cardiovascular disease in the cardiovascular health study, *Am J Epidemiol*, 65, 1, 14-21

Page 54   57 Leung CW et al, 2014, Soda and cell aging: associations between sugar-sweetened beverage consumption and leukocyte telomere length in healthy adults from the National Health and Nutrition Examination Surveys, *Am J Public Health*, 104, 12, 2425-31

Chapter 11

Page 57   58 LeBlanc WE et al, 2009, Formation of hydroxymethylfurfural in domestic high-fructose corn syrup and its toxicity to the honey bee (Apis mellifera), *J Agric Food Chem*, 57, 16, 7369-76

Page 58   59 Zirbes L et al, 2013, Hydroxymethylfurfural: a possible emergent cause of honey bee mortality? *J Agric Food Chem*, 61, 49, 11865-70

         60 http://www.ams.usda.gov/AMSv1.0/getfile?dDocName=STELPR DC5087792

Page 59   61 Lu J et al, 2014, Manuka-type honeys can eradicate biofilms produced by Staphylococcus aureus strains with different biofilm-forming abilities, *PeerJ*, 2, e326

         62 Majtan J, 2011, Methylglyoxal – a potential risk factor of Manuka honey in healing of diabetic ulcers, Evid Based Complement *Alternat Med*, 295494

         63 Molan P, Rhodes T, 2015, Honey: A Biologic Wound Dressing, *Wounds*, 27, 6, 141-51

Page 61   64 Mikkola JP et al, 2003, Hydrogenation of xylose to xylitol on sponge nickel catalyst – a study of the process and catalyst deactivation kinetics, *Braz J Chem Eng*, 20, 3

Page 62   65 Li L, Seeram NP, 2011, Further investigation into maple syrup yields 3 new lignans, a new phenylpropanoid, and 26 other phytochemicals, *J Agric Food Chem*, 59, 14, 7708-16

         66 http://www.uvm.edu/~pmrc/sugarprof.pdf

Page 66   67 http://www.glycemicindex.com/foodSearch.php?num=2659&ak=detail

         68 https://www.tropicaltraditions.com/coconut_palm_sugar.htm

         69 http://www.fao.org/ag/aga/agap/frg/lrrd/lrrd11/1/dali111.htm

Page 67   70 Scheid MM et al, 2014, Freeze-dried powdered yacon: effects of FOS on serum glucose, lipids and intestinal transit in the elderly. *Eur J Nutr* 53, 7, 1457-64

         71 Aybar MJ et al, 2001, Hypoglycemic effect of the water extract of Smallantus sonchifolius (yacon) leaves in normal and diabetic rats. *J Ethnopharmacol*, 74, 2, 125-32

         72 Hill S et al, 2014, The effect of non-caloric sweeteners on cognition, choice and post-consumption satisfaction, *Appetite*, 83, 82-88.

         73 Swithers SE, Davidson RL, 2008, A role for sweet taste: calorie predictive relations in energy regulation in rats, *Behav Neurosci*, 122, 1, 161-73

Page 68   74 Feijo Fde M et al, 2013, Saccharin and aspartame, compared with sucrose, induce greater weight gain in adult Wistar rats, at similar total caloric intake levels, *Appetite*, 60, 1, 203-7

75 Hazuda H et al, presented at the American Diabetes Association's Scientific Sessions, San Diego, 2011

76 Swithers SE, 2013, Artificial sweeteners produce the counterintuitive effect of inducing metabolic derangements, *Trends Endocrinol Metab*, 24, 9, 431-4

77 Suez J et al, 2014, Artificial sweeteners induce glucose intolerance by altering the gut microbiota. *Nature*, 514, 181-186

78 Diamant M et al, 2011, Do nutrient-gut-microbiota interactions play a role in human obesity, insulin resistance and type 2 diabetes? *Obes Rev*, 12, 4, 272-81

79 Cani PD, Delzenne NM, 2009, The role of the gut microbiota in energy metabolism and metabolic disease. *Curr Pharm Des*, 15, 13, 1546-58

Page 69   80 Holton KF et al, 2012, The effect of dietary glutamate on fibromyalgia and irritable bowel symptoms, *Clin Exp Rheumatol*, 30, 6 Suppl 74, 10-7

Page 70   81 Tollefsen KE et al, 2012, Presence, fat and effects of the intense sweetener sucralose in the aquatic environment, *Sci Total Environ*, 438, 510-6

82 Wiklund AK et al, 2012, Sucralose – an ecotoxicological challenger? *Chemosphere*, 86, 1, 50-5)

Chapter 15

Page 92   83 Afkhami-Ardekani M, Shojaoddiny-Ardekani A, 2007, Effect of vitamin C on blood glucose, serum lipids & serum insulin in type 2 diabetes patients, 126, 5, 471-4, *Indian J Med Res.* 2007 Nov;126(5):471-4

Page 93   84 Simopoulos AP, 2011, Evolutionary Aspects of Diet: The Omega-6/Omega-3 Ratio and the Brain, *Mol Neurobiol*, 44, 2, 203-15

85 Yu YH et al, 2011, The function of porcine PPARγ and dietary fish oil effect on the expression of lipid and glucose metabolism related genes, *J Nutr Biochecm*, 22, 2, 179-86

86 Gray B et al, 2013, Omega-3 fatty acids: a review of the effects on adiponectin and leptin and potential implications for obesity management, *Eur J Clin Nutr*, 67, 12, 1234-42

87 Holness MJ et al, 2003, Diabetogenic impact of long-chain omega-3 fatty acids on pancreatic beta-cell function and the regulation of endogenous glucose production, *Endocrinology*, 144, 9, 3958-68

Page 94   88 Ponnampalam EN et al, 2006, Effect of feeding systems on omega-3 fatty acids, conjugated linoleic acid and trans fatty acids in Australian beef cuts: potential impact on human health, *Asia Pac J Clin Nutr*, 15, 1, 21-9

Page 94   89 de Roos NM et al, 2003, Trans fatty acids, HDL-cholesterol, and cardiovascular disease. Effects of dietary changes on vascular reactivity, *Eur J Med Res*, 8, 8, 355-7.

90 Kavanagh et al, 2007, Trans fat diet induces abdominal obesity and changes in insulin sensitivity in monkeys, *Obesity*, 15, 1675-1684

Page 95   91 Yeh,G.Y. Et al, 2003, Systematic review of herbs and dietary supplements for glycemic control in diabetes', *Diabetes Care*, 26, 4, 1277-1294

92 Kozlovsky AS et al, 1986, Effects of diets high in simple sugars on urinary chromium losses, *Metabolism*, 35, 515-8

Page 96   93 A scientific review: the role of chromium in insulin resistance, 2004, *Diabetes Educ*, Suppl 2-14

94 Singer GM, Geohas J, 2006, The effect of chromium picolinate and biotin supplementation on glycemic control in poorly controlled patients with type 2 diabetes mellitus: a placebo-controlled, double-blinded, randomised trial, *Diabetes Technol Ther*, 8, 6, 636-43).

95 Yaqi T et al, 2013, The role of zinc in the treatment of taste disorders, *Recent Pat Food Nutri Agric*, 5, 1, 44-51

96 Chen MD et al, 2000, Zinc may be a mediator of leptin production in humans, *Life Sci*, 66, 22, 2143-9

97 Luong KV, Nguyen LT, 2012, The impact of thiamine treatment in the diabetes mellitus, 4, 3, 153-60, *J Clin Med Res*. 2012 Jun;4(3):153-60. doi: 10.4021/jocmr890w. Epub 2012 May 15

98 Sakakeeny L et al, 2012, Plasma pyridoxal-5-phosphate is inversely associated with systemic markers of inflammation in a population of U.S. adults, *J Nutr*, 142, 7, 1280-5

Page 97   99 Fernandez-Mejia C, 2005, Pharmacological effects of biotin, *J Nutri Biochem*, 16, 7, 424-7

100 Pearce SH, Cheetham TD, 2010, Diagnosis and management of vitamin D deficiency, *BMJ*, 340, 7738, 142-147

Page 98   101 Mitri J et al, 2011, Vitamin D and type 2 diabetes: a systematic review, *European Journal of Clinical Nutrition*, 65, 1005-1015

102 Darup D et al, 2012, A reverse J-shaped association of all-cause mortality with serum 25-hydroxyvitamin D in general practice: the CopD study, *J Clin Endocrinol Metab*, 97, 8, 2644-52

103 Suksomboon N et al, 2011, Effects of vitamin E supplementation on glycaemic control in type 2 diabetes: systematic review of randomized controlled trials, *J Clin Pharm Ther*, 36, 1, 53-63

Page 99   104 Mooren FC, 2015, Magnesium and disturbances in carbohydrate metabolism, *Diabetes Obes Metab*, May 13, ahead of print)

Page 99   105 Hruby A et al, 2014, Higher magnesium intake reduces risk of impaired glucose and insulin metabolism and progression from prediabetes to diabetes in middle-aged Americans, *Diabetes Care*, 37, 2, 419-27

106 Hodgson JM et al, 2002, Coenzyme Q10 improves blood pressure and glycaemic control: a controlled trial in subjects with type 2 diabetes, *Eur J Clin Nutr,* 56, 11, 1137-42

107 Skarlovnik A et al, 2014, Coenzyme Q10 supplementation decreases statin-related mild-to-moderate muscle symptoms: a randomized clinical study, *Med Sci Monit*, 20, 2183-8

108 Cederberg H et al, 2015, Increased risk of diabetes with statin treatment is associated with impaired insulin sensitivity and insulin secretion: a 6 year follow-up study of the METSIM cohort, *Diabetologia*, 58, 5, 1109-7

109 El Midaoui A and de Champlain J, 2002, Prevention of hypertension, insulin resistance and oxidative stress by alpha-lipoic acid, *Hypertension*, 39, 2, 303-7

110 Huerta AE et al, 2015, Effects of α-lipoic acid and eicosapentaenoic acid in overweight and obese women during weight loss, *Obesity* (Silver Spring), 23, 2, 313-21

Page 100 111 Nobre AC et al, 2008, L-theanine, a natural constituent in tea, and its effect on mental state, *Asia Pac J Clin Nutr*, 17, Suppl 1, 167-8

112 Rao TP et al 2015, In Search of a Safe Natural Sleep Aid, *J Am Coll Nutr*, March 11, 1-12, Ahead of print

INDEX

acanthosis nigricans 35

acesulfame-K 68

acetylcholine 42

acrohorda 35

addiction 20, 21, 81, 140

Adrenal Stress Test 50

adrenaline 25, 27, 31, 48, 75, 76, 77, 78

advanced glycation end-products (AGEs) 53, 54, 59

agave 56, 57, 72

ageing 39, 51, 53, 54, 62, 140

aggressive outburst 48

alcohol 15, 56, 60, 61, 68, 71, 77

allergies 48, 97

alpha-lipoic acid 99

Alzheimer's 31, 37, 41, 42, 43, 44, 93, 94

amino acids 66, 68, 69

amyloid 41,

amyloid beta 37, 42, 43, 44

anaerobic glycolysis 45

angiogenesis 45

antioxidants 62, 66, 77, 101

anxiety 22, 48, 51, 100, 101

apoptosis 46

appetite 16, 23, 25, 27, 49, 56, 64, 67, 68, 77, 81, 96

apple shape 26

artificial sweeteners 15, 28, 55, 67, 68, 81, 141

aspartame 68, 69

atherosclerosis 29

auto-immune 37

Ayurvedic 65

B vitamins 32, 64, 65, 66, 88, 96, 100, 142

barley malt extract 63

barley malt syrup 63, 105, 117, 118

beneficial bacteria 66, 67, 68, 88, 89, 131

beta amyloid plaque 41, 42

black strap molasses 60

bloating 60, 62, 89

blood flow 43

blurred vision 36

BMI 36

body fat percentage 25, 67

breast cancer 33, 41, 45, 46

brown rice syrup 63, 126, 131, 134

cacao 101, 102, 112, 123, 126, 129, 133

caffeine 76, 77, 81, 89, 101, 141

calcium 62, 64, 66, 91,

calories 10, 16, 18, 20, 24, 38, 49, 60, 63, 64, 67, 68, 74, 75, 76, 91

cancer 33, 39, 40, 42, 45, 46, 54, 69, 93, 97, 140

cane juice 64, 65

carbohydrate 17, 45, 72, 77, 78, 83, 89, 99, 141

carbohydrates 15, 16, 18, 19, 21, 24, 30, 31, 43, 62, 78, 85, 95, 96

cardiovascular 31

carob 102, 112, 121, 123, 126, 129

caster sugar 15

cephalic phase insulin release 28

cerebellum 42

China 34

chlorella 88

cholesterol 29, 30, 31, 32, 33, 36, 40, 42, 52, 56, 68, 92, 94

chromium 64, 95, 96, 142

chromosomes 54

circadian rhythm 43

clostridium 59

cocoa 101

coconut 65, 66, 85, 86, 87, 101, 106, 107, 110, 119, 121, 122, 123, 124, 125, 128, 130, 131, 134, 139,

coconut blossom syrup 65

coconut nectar 65

coconut palm sugar 65

coconut sugar 65, 66

coconut syrup 65

co-enzyme Q10 99

collagen 53

complex carbohydrates 15

cortisol 25, 26, 27, 31, 43, 44, 45, 48, 49, 50, 51, 52, 75, 77, 78

cravings 10, 27, 67, 74, 77, 78, 81, 83, 95, 96, 99, 141, 142

C-reactive protein 30, 31, 40

dairy foods 30

dandelion 88

dehydroepiandrosterone 50

dementia 41, 42, 43, 94, 97, 140

demerara sugar 15

depression 33, 48, 51, 93, 100

detox 81, 82, 83, 84, 85, 86, 88, 89, 140

dextrose 15, 16, 63, 73

DHEA 50, 52

diabetes 9, 22, 23, 30, 31, 32, 33, 34, 35, 36, 37, 38, 39, 40, 41, 43, 49, 59, 62, 68, 92, 93, 94, 96, 98, 99, 100, 140

diarrhoea 60, 61, 62

diet drinks 68, 76

digestive problems 33, 48

disaccharides 16

dizziness 48

DNA 54

dopamine 67

elastin 53

energy 10, 15, 16, 19, 20, 21, 24, 27, 30, 35, 45, 49, 50, 83, 86, 87, 95, 96, 99, 140

erythritol 15, 61

essential fats 94

evaporated cane juice 64, 65

exercise 46, 75, 79, 82, 83

fasting 40, 75, 76, 92

fasting glucose 38, 39, 53

fat around the middle book 26, 106, 144

fat stores 25

fatigue 36, 48, 50, 75, 93, 99

fatty liver 22, 56, 68

fight or flight response 27

flaxseeds 86, 88, 93, 112, 121, 125

FODMAP diet 60, 62

forgetfulness 48, 93

FOS 66, 67

free radical damage 39

frontal lobe 42

fructooligosaccharide 67

fructose 15, 16, 17, 22, 23, 55, 56, 57, 60, 62, 63, 95

fructose-glucose 17, 22

gestational diabetes 36

ghrelin 25, 56

glucagon 25

glucose 15, 16, 17, 23, 24, 25, 30, 34, 35, 37, 38, 39, 40, 42, 43, 45, 47, 48, 49, 56, 57, 58, 60, 62, 63, 67, 78, 92, 93, 95, 96, 97, 98, 99

glucose intolerance 68

glucose tolerance test 38

glucose-fructose 22, 72

Glycaemic Index 17, 20, 43, 46, 65

glycation 39, 53, 54

glycosylated haemoglobin 39, 46, 53

granulated sugar 15

gut bacteria 68

haemoglobin 39, 54

HbA1c 39, 40, 92, 98,

HDL cholesterol 33, 36, 40

headaches 33, 48, 82, 89

heart disease 9, 23, 29, 30, 31, 33, 51, 54, 56, 68, 93, 94, 97, 100, 140,

high blood pressure 68, 99

high fructose corn syrup 17, 22, 56, 57

hippocampus 42, 43

honey 18, 57, 58, 59, 62

hydrogenation 60, 61

hypoglycaemia 48

hypothalamus 42

IBS 60, 61, 62, 67, 69

icing sugar 15

immune 32, 37, 42, 45, 50, 51, 92, 96, 97

inflammation 10, 17, 30, 31, 32, 33, 43, 54, 81, 93, 94

insomnia 48, 101

insulin 22, 23, 24, 25, 26, 28, 30, 31, 32, 33, 35, 37, 40, 41, 42, 43, 45, 46, 48, 49, 55, 60, 61, 68, 75, 92, 93, 94, 95, 96, 98

insulin receptors 35, 92, 94,

insulin resistance 37, 40, 43, 49, 68, 99

insulin sensitisers 37

irritability 48

irritable bowel syndrome 51, 61

jaggery 64, 65, 112

joint pain 51, 97

lactose 15, 16, 85, 89

LDL cholesterol 33

leptin 23, 25, 56, 96

libido 10

light exposure 44

liver 22, 23, 24, 25, 27, 31, 33, 39, 45, 48, 56, 88

liver disease 33, 56, 68

liver spots 53

low blood sugar 48, 67

l-theanine 99, 100

magnesium 60, 64, 66, 91, 98, 99, 100, 142

maltodextrin 16, 17

maltose 15, 16, 63

manganese 60, 62

Manuka honey 59

maple syrup 62, 67, 76, 102, 103, 104, 111, 112, 113, 114, 116, 120, 123, 124, 125, 127, 131, 132, 139

melatonin 43, 44

metabolic syndrome 40, 68

methylglyoxal 33, 58

Mexico 34, 56

molasses 15, 59, 60, 62, 64

monosaccharides 16

MSG 69

multivitamin and mineral 95, 142

muscle cramps 48

muscle pain 33

muscovado sugar 15

National Diet and Nutrition Survey 11

natural killer cells 45

nervousness 48

obesity 9, 19, 30, 34, 51, 67, 68, 100

omega 3 92, 93, 94, 95

omega 6 93, 94

oral glucose tolerance test 38

organic honey 58

overweight 20, 30, 35, 36, 37, 46, 68

oxidative stress 31, 42

oxygen 42, 45

palm sugar 65, 66

palmyra palm 65

palpitations 48

pancreas 24, 25, 28, 35, 37, 41, 45, 49, 99

PCOS 36

pear shape 26

plaque 29, 31, 41, 42

polyol 15, 60, 61

polyphenols 62, 66

potassium 60, 66

prebiotics 67

prediabetes 34, 35, 36, 39, 43, 99

premature ageing 39, 51, 140

probiotics 16, 88

protein 37, 41, 53, 78, 84, 85, 86, 87, 89, 90, 95, 121, 123, 125, 137, 141 psyllium 88

rapadura 64

receptors 20, 35, 67, 92, 93, 94

rickets 97

saccharin 68, 69

SAD 97

seasonal affective disorder 97

serving size 72

sex drive 48, 51

simple carbohydrates 16

skin 35, 51, 53, 54, 55, 81, 84, 88, 93, 94, 97

skin tags 35, 45

slave trade 13

sleep 10, 25, 33, 44, 50, 51, 81, 82, 100, 140

Soil Association 58

sorbitol 15, 61

statins 32, 33, 99

stevia 63, 64

stress 34, 48, 49, 50, 51, 52, 75, 78, 79, 81, 96, 98, 99, 140

stress hormones 27, 31, 48, 49, 50, 77, 78, 81, 99

stress test 50

strokes 33

sucralose 68, 69, 70

sucrose 15, 16, 22, 23, 55, 60, 62, 63, 68, 69, 95

sugar alcohol 15, 61

sugar beet 14, 15, 70

sugar cane 12, 14, 15, 16, 59, 60, 64, 65, 70

sugar cane juice 59, 65

sugar tax 19

sundowning 43

supplements 16, 22, 56, 91, 93, 95, 142

sweating 48, 84

symptoms of type 2 diabetes 36

table sugar 22, 55, 63

telomeres 54

testing for diabetes 38

testing for insulin resistance 40

theobromine 101

trans fats 94

treacle 15

triglycerides 22, 23, 30, 31, 36, 40, 56

turbinado sugar 15

type 1 diabetes 37

type 2 diabetes 9, 23, 30, 31, 32, 34, 36, 37, 38, 39, 40, 41, 43, 49, 62, 68, 92, 93, 94, 96, 98, 99, 100, 140

type 3 diabetes 37, 41

unconscious eating 79

vascular dementia 41, 42

vitamin A 64

vitamin B12 32, 65

vitamin B6 32, 60, 96

vitamin C 92, 95, 98, 142

vitamin D 97, 98

vitamin E 98

VLDL 31, 40

waistline 16, 68

weight 16, 23, 24, 25, 26, 27, 35, 38, 46, 51, 56, 57, 62, 63, 64, 67, 68, 73, 81, 93, 94, 99, 140,

weight gain 24, 26, 35, 51, 62, 64, 67, 140

whole cane sugar 64

World Health Organisation 18

wrinkles 53, 54

xylitol 15, 60, 61

xylose 60, 61

yacon syrup 66

zinc 62, 64, 66, 91, 96